FABULOUS AT FIFTY & BEYOND

FABULOUS AT FIFTY
& BEYOND

A Complete Guide to Looking and Feeling Your Best

ANGELA RIPPON

MACMILLAN

First published 2003 by Macmillan
an imprint of Pan Macmillan Ltd
Pan Macmillan, 20 New Wharf Road, London N1 9RR
Basingstoke and Oxford
Associated companies throughout the world
www.panmacmillan.com

ISBN 1 4050 3378 9

9 8 7 6 5 4 3 2

A CIP catalogue record for this book
is available from the British Library.

Designed by designsection
Printed and bound in Great Britain
by Butler & Tanner

Contents

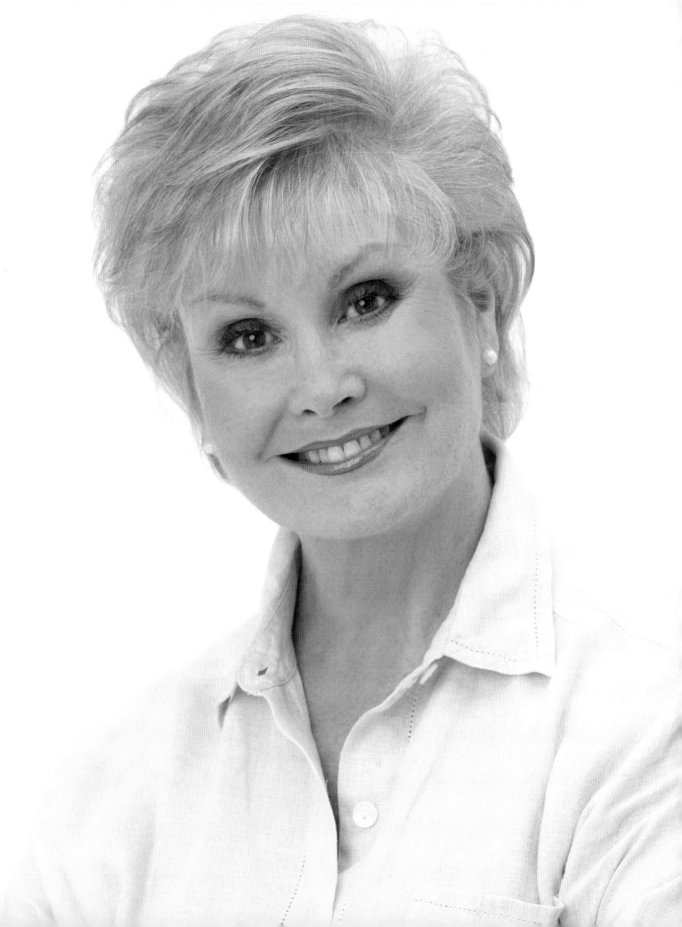

Introduction

My fiftieth birthday was a major turning point for me. As the day grew nearer I was torn between staying quietly at home and pretending this birthday was no different from any other, or throwing a great party for all my friends and celebrating my half century. It was a simple choice: denial or debauchery. No contest really. In the end I went for the party and basked in the glow of all those people who said I didn't look a day over forty-five, and reminded myself that the date was just a mark on the calendar – it didn't have to be a blight on my life; in fact, quite the reverse. With maturity I'd gained wisdom without losing my zest for life and had the freedom, opportunity and fortunately the income to indulge my passion for travel and the self-confidence to know, and be, myself. Cosmetics would help me to continue to look reasonably good, and I had a degree of good health which, aided and abetted by medical science, would ensure I would be fit enough to enjoy my life to the full for a few decades more.

OK, so I have to work at it. Age and gravity leave their marks on the skin, the hair and the body in general, no matter how well you look after them. But these days, hitting fifty and beyond no longer means heading for the rocking chair or checking out of life and leaving all the fun to the thirty-somethings.

Advances in medical science, and the general good health of the nation, means most of us can look forward to living well beyond the biblical three score years and ten. So, with over a third of our lives still stretching ahead of us after fifty, why waste all those years sitting in God's waiting room when there's a world still full of opportunity, challenge and, yes, fun.

Obviously good health and mobility are key factors in getting the most out of our senior years. I remember the best advice I ever had on this front came over thirty years ago from the first of the keep-fit gurus Eileen Fowler. She came to Westward Television in Plymouth where I was working in the 1970s. A petite, sprightly woman in her sixties, she bounced into the studio full of energy and enthusiasm, and demonstrated how fit and agile she was by bending over to touch the floor, then doing a series of high kicks and floor exercises. (Remember, this was *way* before Jane Fonda, Diana Moran the Green

Goddess or any of the television exercise queens were telling us to 'go for the burn'.) Her philosophy was simple. 'Think of the body as a machine,' she said. 'It's full of moving parts that will seize up and rust if you don't keep them well oiled and moving.'

It was sensible, no-nonsense advice and I've followed it all my life. Admittedly I'm not as supple as I was at twenty or thirty, but regular exercise has kept me fit and well. I suppose you could say I'm a bit like a vintage car: I need regular maintenance, but the looks are still reasonable, and everything is still in good working order!

Because I *feel* good about myself, I want to go on *looking* good. With so many cosmetic products designed for mature skins and bodies, never has it been so easy for women (and men) of all ages to beat the clock and maintain their looks, health, energy and sheer joy in life well beyond retirement.

That's what this book is all about: recognizing that fifty is a milestone, but not one that precedes the decline into old age so much as a signal for the start of a terrific new phase of your life. It's a milestone that offers you the opportunity to take a long hard look at your lifestyle to ensure you stay fit, active and healthy enough to enjoy the years approaching retirement, and after, to the full. Compared to our parents and grandparents, our generation, the generation of baby boomers, is healthier, living longer and looking better. With glamorous role models like Joan Collins, Catherine Deneuve and Harrison Ford proving that, like good wine, men and women improve with age, we know we can go on looking terrific, too.

Now, I know not everyone wants to look like a mature model on the front cover of *Vogue* (though I know several women who would look wonderful on the cover of any glossy mag). For the majority of us, our goal is simply to go on making the most of what we've got so we feel good about ourselves. And while every women's magazine in the world is constantly offering advice on beauty and good health, they often overlook the fact that once we hit fifty and beyond, *our* needs and expectations are somewhat different from those we had in our twenties and thirties. Hormonal changes affect our whole body including our skin and our hair: we loose definition and tone; gain wrinkles, grey hair and extra weight; stiffen up, slow down, and find that the make-up colours, textures and techniques that worked in our youth seem less effective on older skin.

So this book is a top-to-toe guide to beauty and health aimed specifically at women (and men) of fifty plus. It gives a wealth of advice, encouragement and information from experts on those things that can make all the difference to your general wellbeing, health and looks for the next thirty years or more.

For instance, during more than a quarter of a century in television I've worked with some of the best make-up artists in the business, and along the way I've picked up all sorts of practical tips and hints. Add to that the knowledge that's come from writing a monthly beauty column for a national magazine, and working with Europe's top cosmetics houses, and I have a store of ideas for cosmetic pampering that really delivers results.

Cosmetic surgery is no longer a whim of the rich and famous. Some procedures are almost as common, and easy, as a manicure. I'll guide you through some of the techniques, and offer you advice on how to get the best results.

But while cosmetic care is a great way of presenting a confident, attractive face to the world, the real key to getting the most out of our mature years lies in enjoying good health and a relatively pain-free existence. So I'll also be examining the principles and rules of maintenance, both mainstream and alternative, that need to be applied to the body as a whole, and its individual parts, to keep it in good working order and to improve vitality.

Exercise is obviously an important part of that goal, and I hope you find the exercises in the final chapter of the book will be of benefit to you, regardless of your age or present state of physical fitness, and will help keep the 'machine' supple and strong. Because I've had so many letters from people asking for help with exercise after hip or knee operations, or to combat arthritic joints, there's a special section on specific problem areas as well.

Exercise, sensible eating patterns, a positive outlook and generally keeping yourself looking and feeling good all go a long way towards ensuring a happy and healthy retirement. But we all recognize things can still go wrong. As the body ages, bits wear out, break down or simply succumb to influences beyond our control. Heart attacks, stroke, rheumatism, arthritis, cancer, cataracts and dodgy hips are just some of the things that could be lurking in the wings as the years advance. I don't know how to prevent any of those things, but I certainly know a lot of people who can help you deal with them, and reduce the risks of them occurring in the first place, so you'll find them listed in this book as well.

In fact, for every subject discussed in this book I've consulted experts who really are leaders in their fields and have added their knowledge and expertise to my own experience.

A friend of mine has a notice in his kitchen that reads, 'After fifty it's all patch, patch, patch.' I don't believe it has to be that way. I'm prepared to work just that little bit harder to maintain my health and vitality so I can cope with whatever life and the Fates throw my way. And because, as it says in the song, 'I enjoy being a girl', I'd like to think that, whatever my age, I will always want to present a well-groomed and confident face to the world. As far as I'm concerned, after fifty, with luck and good health, there's at least a third of my life still to be lived. I don't want to waste one minute of it, and I'm sure you don't either.

I hope that in these pages you'll find some of the inspiration, advice and support that will make *you* feel fabulous at fifty – and beyond.

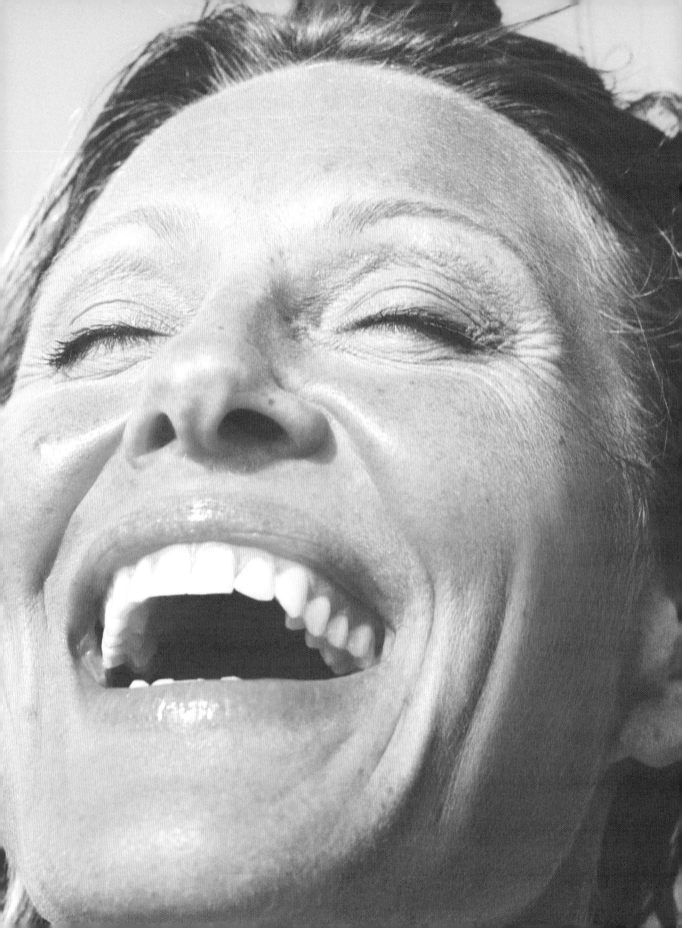

1
THE FACE

There's no getting away from it. Even though we see our faces in a mirror every day of our lives, there suddenly comes a moment when the woman staring back at us no longer looks quite so familiar. 'Hey, what happened to that forty-year-old I used to meet every morning? She's gone, she's changed.' They're probably quite subtle changes too: a few more wrinkles here, a bit more of a sag on the jawline there. Things that have crept up on us when we weren't looking. Things, which frankly, we can do very little to stop.

Regardless of whether we wear make-up or not our face is a map of our whole personality. If we've laughed a lot or frowned too often the evidence is there for all to see, etched on our faces, along with pain and disappointment, rude good health or the debris of too much sun and too many late nights, booze and ciggies.

But another of the great advantages of being a woman in the twenty-first century is that while we might not be able to prevent the march of time across our face, we can slow it down quite a bit and make major improvements in areas that have been previously neglected.

OK, so we can't turn back the clock, and we're never going to look twenty or thirty again. But as mature women we should be confident about the looks we've grown into and aim to maintain a skin that's clear, supple and glowing with good health. That alone will knock off the years and keep people guessing about the date on your birth certificate.

THE FACE
Keeping Young and Beautiful

So let's get the science bit over with first. How does skin 'work' and why does it wrinkle?

To make things easy, think of the skin on your face as a three-layered sandwich (it's a lot more complicated than that, but we're not reading for a degree in epidemiology here, just about youthful good looks). The bottom layer is called the dermis. It's packed full of living cells rich in blood and oxygen which feed the skin. These cells also contain, among other things, natural collagen, the ingredient that gives skin its elasticity. When the dermis is thick and healthy, it acts like a mattress giving firm support to the rest of the skin. The middle layer is called the epidermis. Here, the cells are living off the food provided by the dermis, and producing melanin – a brown pigment that gives skin its colour tone and helps protect it from ultraviolet light. Finally, the top layer, the bit we all see, is known as the stratum corneum.

Think of your skin as being like an escalator in perpetual motion. As the new cells are formed in the dermis, they start to work their way to the surface. Fresh cells are constantly formed below them, pushing them up towards the old cells which are dying off on the surface. The whole process takes between three to four weeks. As the new cells move up through the epidermis they gradually die off, becoming filled with keratin, the tough fibrous protein found in hair and nails, and are almost totally dehydrated.

In youth, the dermis is quite plump and healthy, and the topmost layer fairly thin, but as we age, from about thirty onwards, that situation is reversed: the production of collagen slows down, perhaps your circulation is a bit sluggish and overexposure to the sun and smoking all cause the dermis to get thinner, giving less support and elasticity. That's when fine lines start to deepen into wrinkles because there's no nice plump mattress to support the skin. At the same time cell renewal slows down, and the old skin cells forming the stratum corneum start to accumulate, making the outer layer thicker, so the skin starts to look dull and coarse. Melanin is no longer produced uniformly, and exposure to the sun leads to brown age spots.

So now we know what's happening to our skin. We may not be able to reverse the clock, but we can go some way to reversing the structure. We have to get the 'skin sandwich'

Fruit is an excellent source of vitamin C – one of the ingredients of glowing, healthy and youthful-looking skin.

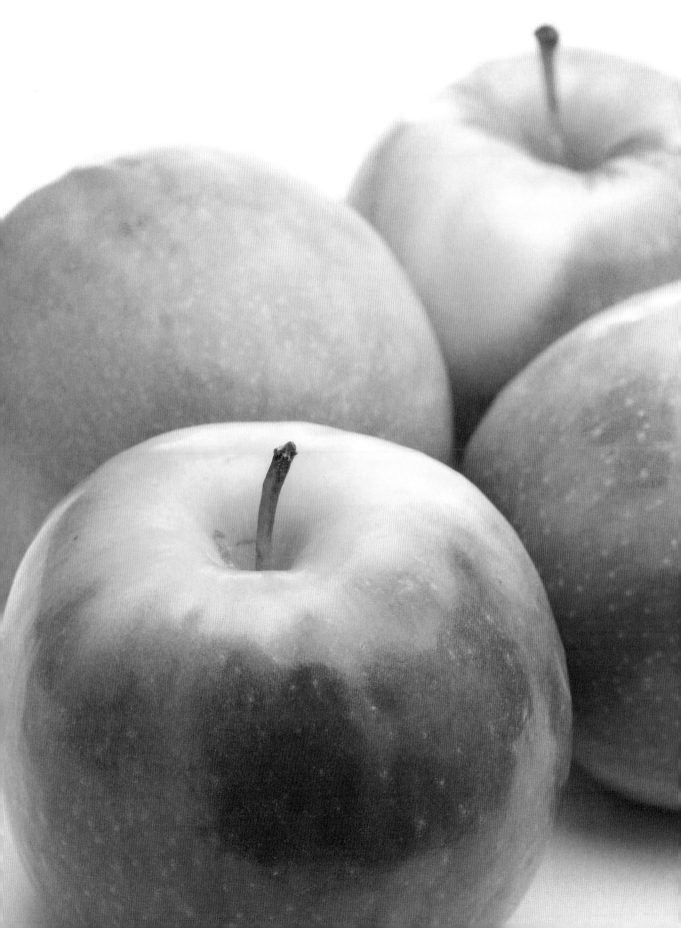

back in balance with a nice thick supporting dermis and a thin stratum corneum.

As with so many really good and effective beauty regimes, we have to start from the inside and work out, so let's begin with your diet. Eat plenty of fresh fruit and vegetables, five to seven servings a day if you can manage it. A healthy, well-balanced diet should provide you with all the proteins, minerals and vitamins – A, B and C – you need and which are essential for healthy skin. You should also include two to three portions of oily fish a week, like herring, mackerel, sardines or salmon, or take a cod liver oil supplement. Oily fish contains omega-3 fatty acids which are good for your skin and for your joints as well. Vitamin E, found in avocado and wheatgerm, or taken as a supplement, will help to rehydrate the skin (see Chapter Eleven).

Drink lots of pure still water, not fizzy. It's carbon dioxide that makes the bubbles in 'sparkling' water, and that's what we breathe out – the body's exhaust fumes. The body needs at least 1.5 litres (about eight glasses) of water a day to keep it well hydrated (see pages 80–2). Water not only hydrates the skin, helping to plump it up, it also flushes out toxins and waste material, keeping the skin clean and healthy from the inside.

Exercise. If you don't have a regular regime (see Chapter Thirteen) take a brisk walk a couple of times a week, or bop around the house to music on the radio. Anything that gets the blood moving, and brings colour to your cheeks is good for you. It's a sign the blood is bringing oxygen and food to the cells in the dermis helping to keep them fit and well nourished. When you apply any creams to your face, give yourself a mini-massage at the same time. It will be another way of boosting the circulation. Patting the skin briskly but gently works particularly well.

Now let's tackle the bit we can see – the stratum corneum.

Cleanse and Exfoliate

Every beautician you speak to will tell you that keeping the skin really clean is the most important part of your routine. When you were young and reckless it might have been OK to occasionally slip into bed in the small hours without removing your make-up after a great night out – but not any more. If you're going to get the stratum corneum back to a nice thin layer, cleansing alone won't be enough. You have to exfoliate regularly – that means at least once a week – to slough off the top thick layer of dead skin cells.

Many skin-care companies make exfoliating washes that are nice and gentle on the skin. They take off the dead cells without scratching the healthy surface or causing irritation. I've found the Cuticura Daily Foaming Face Wash particularly gentle, but my favourite exfoliant is ordinary household salt. I discovered this at the Shrubland Health Spa, where they rub salt all over the body after a sauna. It makes the skin feel like silk – but go steady. I usually lather my face first with a soapless face wash, and then take a handful of salt and rub it in with the wash. Whatever you use, avoid the eyes, but massage the exfoliant all over the face and into all the nooks and crannies, especially around the nose, the chin and the outside of the lips. And don't forget your neck! When you rinse off, your skin should feel really smooth and look radiant and clear. Done regularly on neglected skin it will really make a difference to its texture and appearance. Believe me, it's never too late to start, and within weeks you should see a glowing new you.

Cleansing the face should be done every morning, and without fail every night, regardless of whether you wear make-up or not.

If you use soap, remember the skin is naturally slightly acidic, whereas soap tends to be alkaline, cancelling out the skin's natural acidity. To avoid this, use a soap with a pH level of 5 to 5.6 and make sure you rinse thoroughly.

My own preference is for Liz Earle's Cleanse & Polish (see back of book for mail order details), which removes every scrap of make-up – even stubborn mascara residue – and is removed with a muslin washcloth wrung out in warm water. This gently exfoliates the skin on a daily basis. It's definitely one of My Top Ten Must Haves in my beauty basket (see page 203).

Tone

Cleansing creams do a great job in dissolving make-up and removing surface grime, but always finish with a mild toner to remove any excess grease from the skin before applying moisturizer.

I have to admit that for years I thought the toning part of the beautician's mantra of 'cleanse, tone, moisturize' was a bit of a waste of time. Not any more. Swipe a cotton-wool pad soaked in toner over your face and neck, especially behind the ears and under the hairline, and you'll be amazed at the muck it finds, even on what you might have thought was well-cleansed skin. Some of it will be accumulated grime from the day, the rest is dead skin cells and excess sebum, the skin's natural lubricant. The toner compliments your cleansing routine and tightens up the pores, which in turn will make the surface of the skin less coarse. Look for a toner that has no alcohol in it, as that can be very drying on mature skin. I like L'Oréal's Age Perfect Smoothing Toner, while one of my closest friends swears by good old-fashioned rose water, and she has lovely skin.

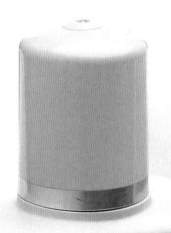

INSTANT BOOST
SKIN TONIC™

NATURALLY ACTIVE INGREDIENTS

ORGANIC ALOE VERA, CALENDULA,
ROSE-SCENTED GERANIUM,
CUCUMBER AND NATURAL VITAMIN E

*Revitalises, soothes and tones
for instant radiance*

NATURALLY ACTIVE
SKINCARE
LIZ EARLE

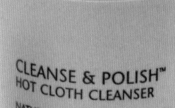

CLEANSE & POLISH™
HOT CLOTH CLEANSER

NATURALLY ACTIVE INGREDIENTS
ALMOND MILK, ROSEMARY,
CHAMOMILE AND EUCALYPTUS
ESSENTIAL OIL

*Cleanses and gently exfoliates
for smoother, clearer skin*

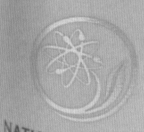

NATURALLY ACTIVE
SKINCARE
LIZ EARLE

Moisturize

Whatever else you may let slip out of your regular beauty routine, never stop using moisturizer on your face. Like me you've probably read articles by 'experts' who say moisturizing creams are a great con and healthy skin doesn't need any extra moisture. Well, that might be just about OK if you're in your twenties, but in your fifties and beyond, nothing could be further from the truth. As we get older, our skin gets naturally drier from within as the collagen production slows down. That stratum corneum gets thicker as the dehydrated cells build up on the surface of the skin like a pile of dry old carpet tiles. Exfoliation will gently scour away the top layer of dead cells, but what's left underneath still needs help. So if you want dull, lifeless, parched skin, then go ahead and ignore moisturizers, but if you want your skin to look fresh, smooth, dewy and healthy, you have to put back some of the moisture that's been leached out by age and the environment. It's especially important to moisturize at night, as it's during the wee small hours, when we're physically at rest, that the body is able to concentrate on cell renewal.

Moisturizers worn during the day will hydrate the skin and protect it against environmental damage. Make sure the one you use includes a SPF (sun protection factor) of at least 15 to shield you against sun damage. Research suggests that over 70 per cent of the damage done to skin by the sun is the result of incidental exposure (like shopping, walking the dog, gardening) rather than the time spent actually lying out and sun bathing.

Moisturizers worn overnight can work when the skin is at its most receptive and cell renewal at its most active. You may be fast asleep, but your skin cells are partying on a cocktail of ingredients to help fight wrinkles and brighten your complexion.

Dr Ian White, consultant dermatologist at St Thomas' Hospital in London, has no interest in cosmetics at all; his concern is healthy skin. This is how he explains the necessity for moisturizing: 'Think of the outer cells of your skin as being like a series of small sponges. When they're sitting on the side of the bath starved of water, they go hard and dry. But the minute you introduce them to the water, they swell up and become soft and pliable. So the most important part of moisturizing is adding moisture – getting the dry, parched cells of the stratum corneum to soak up some water. Then you need to plug the entrances of the cells with a cream or emollient of some sort to keep the water in.'

Simple! And his advice? 'Use glycerine and rose water. It's the only combination you need.'

So where does that leave the multi-million-pound cosmetics industry that spends a small fortune on developing, and then advertising, moisturizers made especially for mature skins? Well, if you look at the list of ingredients, you'll find every moisturizing cream without exception contains water and glycerine. So no change there.

An effective moisturizing regime is key to terrific skin health.

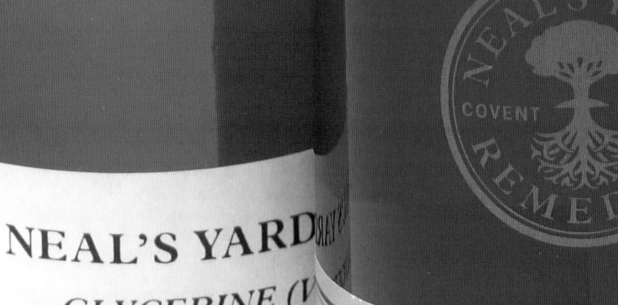

NEAL'S YARD

GLYCERINE (V

INGREDIENTS: GLYCERO

100 ml BN: 0912

LONDON WC2H 9DH www.

NEAL'S
COVENT GA
REMED

ROSEWATE
FOR NORMAL SK

PURE ROSE ABSOLUTE, RENOWNED FOR IT
PROPERTIES AND FOR HELPING TO MAINT
MOISTURE BALANCE, IS MIXED WITH WATE
FRAGRANT SKIN TONER. USE AFTER CLEANSIN
E SKIN. MAY ALSO BE USED TO REFRESH TH

INGREDIENTS: WATER (AQUA), ROSE (ROSA
POLYSORBATE-20, PHENOXYETHANOL

As for the rest of the ingredients, according to Dr White they may all amount to nothing more than a promise in a pot (you'd expect that from a man!). But I'm not convinced. A layer of glycerine on the skin may be fine if you don't want to wear make-up, but if you do, then it's not much use as the make-up will just slide off.

The multi-ingredients in cosmetics-house moisturizers bring extra properties to the skin, not just by providing a good base for make-up but also by soothing and refining it and creating a protective layer against sun and environmental damage. And let's face it, every woman wants to believe the promise on the label. The psychological effect of using some creams can be just as effective in boosting self-confidence and morale as they are in moisturizing the skin. So my advice is to find a cream you like and can afford which suits your skin and use it every morning and evening. You'll feel good about yourself knowing you're doing something that will really make a difference to your appearance, and the glow of self-confidence you'll get from that is something you won't find in any pot.

> Remember – young skin is healthy. Healthy skin looks younger.

Wrinkles

There's no getting away from it. The sun does more damage to your skin, and is more responsible for the formation of wrinkles than any other factor in your life. Talk to any skin specialist, medical or cosmetic, and they'll all say the same thing. Protect your skin from the sun, and you'll increase your chances of keeping your skin healthy and ageless, and decrease the chances of wrinkling up like an old prune (see Sun Damage, page 93).

One of my closest friends has an allergy associated with sunlight, so she never exposes herself to the sun and as a result has fabulous skin with hardly a line on it. I say 'hardly' because even she won't totally escape getting wrinkles, though they'll probably be pretty faint.

It's almost impossible to avoid getting wrinkles somewhere on your face and neck as you get older, simply because they contain some of the most mobile and overworked muscles in the body. If you shrieked at the first sign of a wrinkle, it was more than likely at the corners of your eyes. There are hundreds of tiny muscles around the eye socket, constantly working away every time you blink, laugh, or screw up your face. This means the skin on the surface is forever being stretched and creased into the tiniest of lines, which

Even a top dermatologist recommends rosewater and glycerine – fundamental to all moisturizing potions – as the basic tools for bringing moisture to the skin and keeping it there.

My Fab Four Moisturizers
L'Oréal Age Perfect Day Moisturizer
Neal's Yard Frankincense Nourishing Cream
Liz Earle's Skin Repair
Prescriptives Super Line Corrector

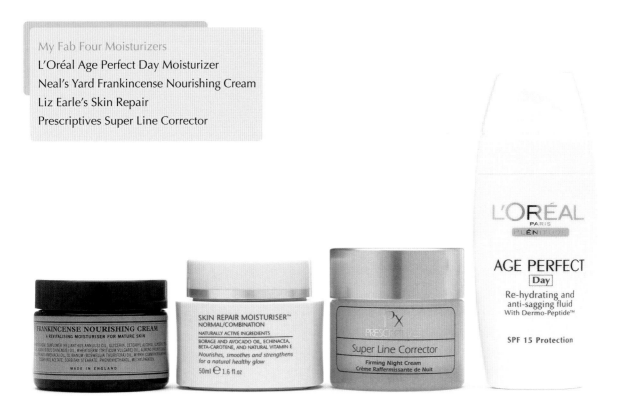

get deeper and more pronounced as your skin dries out and the collagen levels drop, reducing elasticity and removing the firm base which kept everything supported. Over time, the same will happen around your mouth, on either side of your nose, on your forehead and, gradually, over the whole of your face and neck. In every area where the muscles are constantly moving and stretching you have the potential for wrinkles.

The Duchess of Windsor famously always lit her dining room with candles. She reckoned the light they shed was kinder to women's complexions than electric light and made wrinkles less obvious! (And she was right.)

Once established wrinkles are impossible to remove. Surgery can reduce them quite dramatically in some cases (see pages 132–6) but that can be both painful and expensive.

The alternative is first to slow down their progress from fine lines to deep furrows and then, as they say in all the adverts for 'mature skin' moisturizers, 'reduce the appearance' of those lines that are established.

Slowing down their progress can be achieved with a good diet and drinking plenty of water. But the two most important things you can do for your skin are, first, give up smoking (if you haven't already) because smoke is full of pollutants and free radicals which do serious damage to the skin and, second, stay out of the sun! (See Sun Damage, page 93.) Ultraviolet light is the main cause of wrinkles and damaged skin on most women, so wear a hat, and cover your face and neck in at least factor 15 sun cream, or a cosmetic foundation that contains a sunscreen.

Afro-Caribbean skins have so much natural protection against the sun that UV damage leading to wrinkles is less likely. It's loss of collagen that produces wrinkles on black skin, so moisturizing and following a good skin-care regime is an essential first step to slowing down the ageing process.

Reducing the appearance of lines once they're formed means continuing the slowing down regime but, in addition, ensure you regularly cleanse, tone, exfoliate and moisturize. That way you keep the skin hydrated from inside and out, clear away the debris of grime and old skin cells and allow the new, plumper cells to expand, fill up the cracks and even out the appearance of the skin.

And remember – don't stop at the jaw. Always treat the neck as part of the face and take all treatments down over the throat to the collarbone. The skin on the neck is finer than on the face; that's why once it starts to dry out it forms the tiny ridges on the neck we refer to as crêpe.

One final thought: if we all lived our lives never being exposed to the sun, never smoking, laughing, worrying or frowning, totally free from stress and being pampered throughout the day, there's a pretty good chance our faces would stay line free and serene throughout our lifetime. It's also odds on that we'd be the most boring person on the planet. So it's no contest really. Get a life. Get a few wrinkles. But don't let them get out of control.

Three buzzwords have entered the language of skin health and beauty and crop up in every article about anti-ageing, they are free radicals and antioxidants. You can't have one without the other – and this is what they are.

Free radicals are highly unstable molecules, which are able to break down and destroy living cells. They're triggered into action as the result of overexposure to the sun, pollution, cigarette smoke and, in some cases, stress. They attack the DNA in our skin and affect the body's natural repair mechanisms. The older we get, the weaker our defences become and the free radicals home-in on soft targets like collagen and elastin production. Once they've knocked out the manufacturing base, wrinkles and sagging skin are the result. That's why we need front-line support from antioxidants that occur naturally in vitamins A (beta-carotene), C and E, as well as in ginkgo biloba, selenium (see page 154) and green tea. They counter-attack the effects of free radicals, helping to boost and support the body's natural defences against damage and ageing. They can also provide extra protection against environmental damage, especially from the sun, when used in skin-care products.

The letters AHA and BHA appear on many skin preparations promising to 'refresh and renew' your skin.

AHA stands for alpha hydroxy acids, which are usually fruit based and used as exfoliators to loosen and shed dead skin to reveal a fresher, smoother and brighter complexion. They can also help your skin retain moisture and encourage cell renewal. What they won't do is get rid of wrinkles.

Because some people with fair or sensitive skins react badly to AHAs, the gentler BHAs, or beta hydroxy acids, are becoming more popular and more generally used. The most common BHA is salicylic acid, which comes from the bark of the willow tree and has been used for years as an exfoliator.

What you *must* remember is that each of them has the word acid in its name and they can be harmful if misused, so *never* take them for granted. Do a patch test on the delicate skin on the inside of your arm before using any product containing AHAs or BHAs. If you register any itching, redness, soreness or allergic reactions to the product, do not use it.

Face Savers

Need a little help in the fight against wrinkles and poor skin texture? Then you might like to try:

- *Facials* Put your face in the hands of a beauty therapist from time to time. It's a great way of giving yourself and your skin a treat. They offer a range of treatments from steaming to massage, exfoliating and beauty masks. Your skin will be revitalized, and you'll feel terrific after an hour's pampering.

- *Cayci treatment* A method of stimulating the muscles in the face using a series of mild electrical pulses. Done regularly, the skin looks brighter and firmer. It's especially effective around the eye sockets and across the jaw.

- *Acupuncture* I've been having acupuncture on my face for over a year now. The fine needles are placed at specific points on the brow above the eyebrows, on the side of the nose, at each side of the mouth and along the jawline. This helps stimulate and strengthen the muscles and improve the blood flow, giving a firm outline to the face. It's honestly not painful – there's just a faint stinging sensation as the needle is inserted and after that, complete relaxation.

- *Face packs* Such an easy treatment to give yourself at home and guaranteed to brighten up the dullest complexion. If possible, choose a time when you can have a good long soak in the bath to open up the pores or, if that's not possible, prepare your face with a hot flannel before applying the pack. They all contain properties that draw out impurities and shrink the pores. Try to relax while it's working on your face rather than dashing around doing other things. Rinse off with a flannel to make sure you remove all traces of the pack, and then slap on a moisturizer. Result – a glowing complexion that looks clear and feels wonderfully fresh.

• *Exercise* Flabby muscles anywhere on the body lead to flabby, sagging skin as the support system is eroded. Clothes are a great cover-up for the body, but on the face, you're pretty much exposed. So keep the muscles firm and toned to help hold everything together.

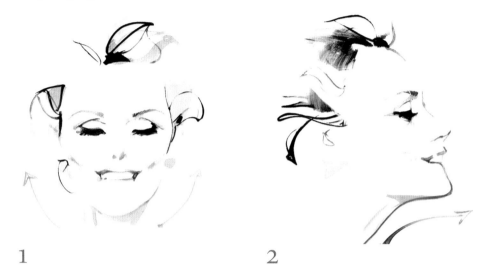

1   2

Try this to keep the jaw and neck muscles toned.

1 Draw your lower lip over your lower teeth and pull back the corners of your mouth into a strong grin exposing your upper teeth (you should already feel the muscles working).

2 Keeping your lip over your teeth, push your jaw forward, then bring it back, really making the muscles in your jaw and neck work hard. Repeat ten times, twice a day. It takes only seconds to do, but as the muscles get stronger you should notice a real change in the outline of your profile.

Surgical Solutions

Cosmetic surgery and anti-ageing treatments are fast becoming the preferred and accepted way for thousands of women to roll back the years. Cutting, lifting, peeling or injecting are now all perfectly acceptable routes to follow if you want to remove wrinkles and rejuvenate skin. And what's more, you can now do it without being labelled vain, paranoid or egotistical. You're just doing what a girl has to do to keep her looks and feel good about herself (see Chapter Nine).

Unwanted Hair

Hormonal changes associated with the menopause can often produce extra facial hair in some women. It may be soft and downy, like the hair on a peach, or start sprouting in coarse individual hairs especially around the chin.

- *Bleaching* is probably the easiest and most effective way of dealing with the soft down that usually appears on the cheeks and chin, and the faint 'moustache' on the upper lip. If you wear make-up, try to avoid using loose powder, which clings to the fine hairs and makes them look more obvious. Instead, go for an all-in-one foundation which will give a matt finish to the skin, making the hairs less noticeable.
- *Waxing* is a really efficient way of removing hair from legs and arms, but don't be tempted to use wax on the upper lip. It tends to be much too aggressive on mature skin and can even rip the skin itself causing great discomfort and damage. That's one of the reasons why so many facial-hair products carry the warning: 'Not suitable for the elderly or diabetics.' How do you assess 'elderly'? Frankly, age has got nothing to do with it. It's a general precaution, because if your skin is at all slack or very fine, as older skin can be, then you run a real risk of damaging it when you rip off the wax strips. If your skin is still pretty firm, then you should be all right. But, anyway, you're better off using the specially formulated Facial Strips made by Jolen, because they contain no wax at all. They use 'glue', rather like a very strong Sellotape – so much kinder to your skin. Make sure your skin is pulled taut when you apply the strips, and keep it taut when you rip them off. Do it quickly to to avoid the 'ouch' factor, and the hairs should be pulled out of their follicles in one movement. It works particularly well on stubborn upper-lip hair and will give you smooth, hair-free skin for a couple of weeks. Done regularly this will help to weaken the roots so that eventually the hairs will grow much finer and perhaps even disappear altogether. Make sure you finish off with a mild antiseptic cream or lotion, like tea tree oil, to cut down the risk of breaking out in small spots around the area. There's not much point in swapping excess hair for an attack of zits! The downside of 'stripping' is that the hair needs to be long enough for the glue to grip to be effective, so between sessions you will need to use bleach to disguise the growth.
- *Hair-removing creams* also often carry the warning that they're not to be used 'by the elderly or diabetics'. The one exception is made by Boots and is ultra gentle. Used

Experiment with make-up. Have fun with it in the privacy of your own bathroom, or take advantage of the free make-overs offered by cosmetics companies in many department stores. Once you find a look that suits you and gives you confidence, just feeling good about yourself will knock years off your age.

strictly according to the instructions it will remove unwanted hair on the face, leaving your skin silky smooth. But you must do a patch test on the skin of your inner arm to ensure that you have no allergic reaction to the cream before you start.

- *Electrolysis* is the permanent way to remove hair. A fine needle is inserted into individual hair follicles, and a small electric current is passed through the needle to kill the root. It may take several sessions to rid your face of excess hair, as the roots are pretty obstinate and don't always give up at the first shot. The treatment can be quite painful and should only ever be carried out by a qualified professional. Get it wrong and you could suffer infection, even scarring. But when done properly it is permanent – eventually!

- *Laser hair removal* works particularly well on coarse, dark hair and lighter skin tones. The laser heats the base of the hair, killing it without damaging the surrounding skin. About 60 per cent of the hair is removed during each treatment and it may take more than one session to completely remove the excess, as hair grows in cycles. It's a completely safe procedure, but I would advise that laser removal should only ever be done by a skin specialist or a cosmetic surgeon.

- *Individual hairs* that sprout on chins or cheeks can be coarse and stubborn. The simplest way of dealing with them is to get a magnifying mirror, good tweezers and strong daylight. It's not true that plucked hairs grow back thicker and stronger. You'll eventually weaken them and, over time, they'll become less of a problem. If you have hairs growing out of a mole, it's quite safe to pluck them out without doing any damage to the mole.

Make-up

When I was about eight or nine there was a fad at school for autograph books in which we wrote little poems and homilies before signing our names. The only one I remember from that period is:

Little bits of powder,
Little bits of paint,
Make a girl's complexion
Look what it ain't.

Too right! Make-up is the perfect camouflage to cover a multitude of sins, create the illusion of a fresh, glowing complexion, and give a boost to your self-confidence whatever your age or the state of your skin.

Don't be afraid to pick the brains of department-store beauticians. But also don't ever be bullied or persuaded into buying something just because the assistant gets persistent with the sales pitch. Take any samples on offer, consult more than one beautician, then go home and think about your potential purchase. Buy only when you are totally confident and convinced that the product, colour or look is right for you.

Remember, beauty comes from inner confidence, not from all the unused, unwanted, unsuitable pots and tubes you've thrown in a drawer.

Prepare

The great American make-up guru Bobbi Brown believes the best way to prepare your skin before applying any type of foundation is to use a concealer to cover dark circles and imperfections. Creamy, yellow-toned concealers are best and can be used not only on the dark circles under your eyes (see page 52), but also to cover prominent age spots and lighten some of the shadows caused by the deep furrows that run from nose to mouth. Pat the concealer into the skin rather than rub, as it's prone to slide off.

Foundation

This should never be darker or lighter than your natural skin tone, and should only be thick enough to give a dewy, even finish to your complexion. It should leave your skin looking smooth, flawless and perfectly natural, and never be so heavy that it becomes a mask, unlike in the seventeenth and eighteenth centuries when women (and men) wore make-up so toxic and thick, it often cracked off and bits fell into their food or onto their clothes. Yuck.

Foundations that contain built-in moisturizers and light-diffusing particles, like the ones made by L'Oréal and Prescriptives, are perfect for older skins. If you want a light 'hardly there' finish, go for a tinted moisturizer. It won't give you a great deal of coverage, but if you want a natural, sporty look, or are not that keen on wearing make-up at all, they're ideal. They are also perfect for older, heavily lined faces. In our seventies and eighties, if our skins are etched with wrinkles, we have to avoid anything that will clog or puddle in the creases. A tinted moisturizer works because it will give a lovely soft look to the complexion and even out the skin tones without ever giving you a 'made-up' look.

To get the right shade for your skin, do a patch test along your jawbone where your true skin tone will be at its purest. Remember that the lighting in many department stores is often quite harsh and always artificial so, if possible, try and get to some daylight before making your final choice. Yellow tones that give warmth to the complexion look better on mature skin than pinky shades, but getting a good look at the colour in daylight will make it obvious which shade to go for.

A good loose powder keeps foundation fixed and prevents excess sheen. For my skin I've not been able to better Corn Silk.

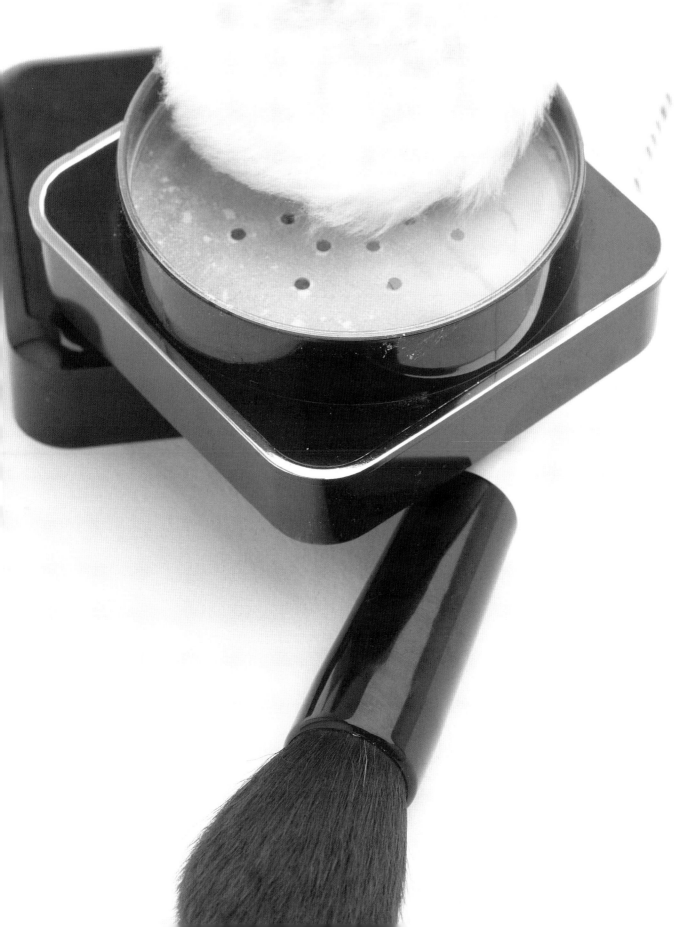

Applying Foundation

Apply foundation in a good light where you can see you're getting an even coverage. I have a magnifying mirror in the bathroom which highlights every lump, bump and imperfection, but gives me a really good view of exactly what I'm putting on my face, and how well it's doing the job.

Some people like to use small sponges to spread the foundation. They certainly give a nice even coverage, but you will waste a lot of make-up because some of it stays in the sponge.

Caroline Barnes, who's one of Britain's leading make-up artists and advises L'Oréal on their cosmetics range, says, 'You can't beat your own fingers.' She recommends you start with clean hands and rub your fingers together to get them slightly warm. This makes it easier to work the foundation into your skin and blend the edges away to nothing. Dot the foundation over the areas you want to cover and then gently work it into your skin. During the day, to give a natural look, you may only want to cover your forehead, nose, cheeks and chin, blending away to nothing from the middle patch before you reach your hairline. For the evening, you'll get a more glamorous look with total coverage, but still keep it light and natural looking. When you come to the bits where you have concealer, pat the foundation into your skin so you keep the lightening effect without wiping it away.

Take the colour just over your jawbone so you're not left with a tide mark, and blend the foundation into the area of your neck immediately below your chin. That spot is often a lot lighter than your face, so you need the foundation to ensure that when people look at you head on, your face and neck match in tone and texture.

If your ears are slightly red, which can happen in older women, swipe a small amount of foundation over the lobes to even up the colour.

And don't forget that throughout the year your skin colour changes from summer to winter, so don't expect the same colour foundation to last all year round.

Powder

The main function of powder is to keep foundation in place and give a soft, matt finish to the skin, especially if your skin has a tendency to be slightly oily.

Loose powder will give you a light finish if you apply it with a soft powder puff or cotton-wool pad and then whisk away the excess with a big, fat powder brush. One of the best loose powders I've found is called Corn Silk. It gives a wonderful translucent finish, and its superfine texture is perfect for mature skins as it doesn't clog the pores and facial lines. It's stocked by Boots and Superdrug but if you have difficulty finding it

If you use a sponge to spread your foundation you'll get good coverage – but a lot will get absorbed into the sponge.

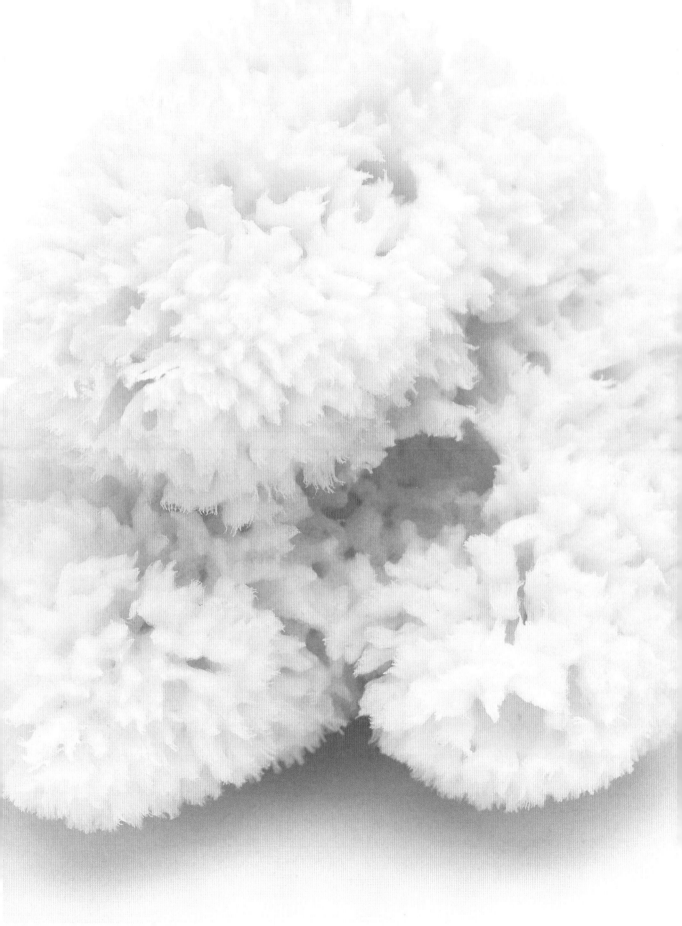

call 01256 844 144. When I'm working in a studio where the lights are unforgiving, or when I'm doing a major presentation, I find I need to make sure my make-up stays matt and fresh for hours, so I load a cotton-wool pad with powder, and press it into my skin. I use quite a lot and leave it there for a few minutes to 'soak' into the foundation (it's a good job no one can see me because I look like I've been hit in the face with a flour bag!). Then, using a large powder brush, I sweep away the excess, leaving a finish that isn't heavy or clogged, but which I know will last without having to be constantly 'touched up'. Now, this is not a routine you'd want to follow if you're aiming for a fresh-looking daytime make-up, but if you've got a big night out or a special event coming up, it will certainly help keep your make-up in place and looking good. I picked up another useful tip from Val Sparkes, who's worked in television make-up for years and was the regular senior stylist on Gloria Hunniford's Channel 5 show. After she's applied powder and blusher, she wrings out a natural sponge in cold water and gently presses it all over the face. This soaks up excess powder and helps to 'set' the foundation in place. The result is a make-up job that survives the heat of the studio lights and gives a lovely natural glow to the skin.

If your skin is very dry, or lined, then you should either use very little powder or avoid it altogether because it will clog in the crevices, drawing attention to wrinkles. Also, don't use powder on skin that has a light covering of 'down'. The powder will cling to the hairs and make them even more noticeable (see Unwanted Hair, page 24).

Pressed Powder
This is best used for lightly touching up if your nose or cheeks start to glow. Try to keep a small face brush with you to whisk away the excess, because sometimes constantly dabbing at your face can lead to a build-up that will make your skin look dry and powdery.

In fact, you might find it better to avoid pressed powder altogether and instead blot your face gently with a tissue to take off the excess oil and shine.

Blusher
The great face-saver and instant pick-me-up. A whisk of blusher across your cheeks can brighten your face and make you look positively radiant even on those days when you might be feeling less than bright eyed and bushy tailed. As mature skin tends to lose colour with age, a blusher should be an essential addition to your make-up kit.

If you've never used blusher before, don't be afraid of it. We're not talking old-fashioned rouge here – those blotches of red on your cheeks that make you look like a Dutch doll. Modern blushers do what it says on the packet: they make your skin glow with health as it would if you were blushing naturally. Mature skins look good with peachy or apricot shades which blend with your own skin tones and don't look like a streak of colour slashed across your face.

Blushers often come packed with their own tiny brush inside a compact. My advice? Throw the brush away; it's next to useless. What you need to give a really natural look is a nice full, round brush. Fill it with colour, give it a good blow to get rid of the excess, then lightly sweep onto the 'apple' of your cheek and up across your cheekbone towards the hairline. Blend it well so you don't see the edges. If you're not sure exactly where to place the powder, grin into the mirror and, where the cheeks form a round cushion, that's where you apply the blusher.

THE FACE
Keeping Healthy

Healthy skin tends to be clean skin. If you follow a regular programme of cleanse, exfoliate, tone and moisturize you're already doing a pretty good job of keeping the topmost layer of skin in a healthy condition. Mature skin has a tendency to become coarse, with open pores that can lead to blackheads, and a complexion that looks grey and lifeless.

You need to improve your general circulation with gentle, daily exercise, and stimulate the circulation of your face with massage. A steam treatment will help to open up and clean out the pores, and regular exfoliation should improve the texture of the skin and prevent the formation of blackheads.

Thread Veins

Those tiny little red veins that usually creep all over the cheeks (though they can appear on the nose and legs) are most likely to be the result of overexposure to the sun and severe weather conditions as the skin gets thinner with age, though hormonal changes, taking HRT, drinking alcohol and smoking can all aggravate them. If they are really fine, foundation will usually camouflage them, and if you make sure to protect your skin with sun lotion or barrier creams, that should stop them getting any worse. But if they really are unsightly and you can't bear to live with them, consult your doctor about the possibility of laser removal. A strong burst of light is used to zap the veins, which then slowly fade and

eventually disappear. There are no needles or incisions, just the sensation of a small pinch on the skin as the laser is applied. You may get a degree of redness and swelling immediately after the treatment, and in some cases the after-effects can be quite painful, but this will fade within a few days. The session can last between fifteen and twenty minutes and the veins should be gone forever.

Alternatively you could consider sclerotherapy, in which an irritant solution is injected directly into the blood vessel so its walls stick together. An anaesthetic cream is applied half an hour before the treatment to dull the pricking sensation you will get from the needle, which is no wider than a human hair. After the injection gentle pressure is applied to the spot. The chemical then spreads through the tiny network of veins which, over the next few weeks, shut down and disappear. For a few days afterwards you may be left with small bumps over the treated area, but these will also soon disappear. A good surgeon will warn you that while thread, or 'spider', veins should fade after one treatment, sclerotherapy is rarely completely effective and you should be prepared to be asked to return for reassessment and possible repeat treatment after about six weeks.

Moles and Melanoma

We all have moles somewhere on our bodies, and for the most part they're pretty harmless. In fact, women with tiny spots on their cheeks or close to the sides of their mouths like Cindy Crawford are usually proud of their 'beauty spots', which can look really attractive.

I had one on my right cheekbone and used to colour it in with brown eye pencil to make it even more distinctive. Then, in my late thirties, it began to change in shape and size, and started to feel tender to the touch. That's when I became aware of how easy it is for a 'beauty spot' to turn into a 'problem spot' and had it removed!

Excessive sun exposure tends to be the trigger that can turn a dormant mole into a potentially malignant melanoma, though there may be other reasons. The signs to look for are these:

- A mole tends to be flat, round or oval and no larger than the diameter of the end of a pencil.
- A melanoma will have irregular edges and can be any colour including tan, brown, pink and especially black.
- A melanoma may be scaly or flaky, ooze or bleed and have a small, open sore that will not heal. The centre may also form a hard lump. They will often itch, and be painful or tender to the touch.

So if you have a mole that suddenly changes shape and colour, or acquire a spot that displays any of the above symptoms, consult your doctor immediately.

If treated in the early stages, a melanoma is easy to cure. Ignored, it will potentially allow the cancer-forming cells to spread to other parts of the body. Australians have been aware for many years of the huge risks posed by unprotected overexposure to the sun. As a result, they've dramatically reduced the number of skin-cancer deaths in their country. Here in Britain, our statistics have gone the other way. More than 8,000 people in the UK die of malignant melanoma every year, and the figures are still rising. So enjoy the sun on your skin, but make sure yours is a healthy, safe exposure.

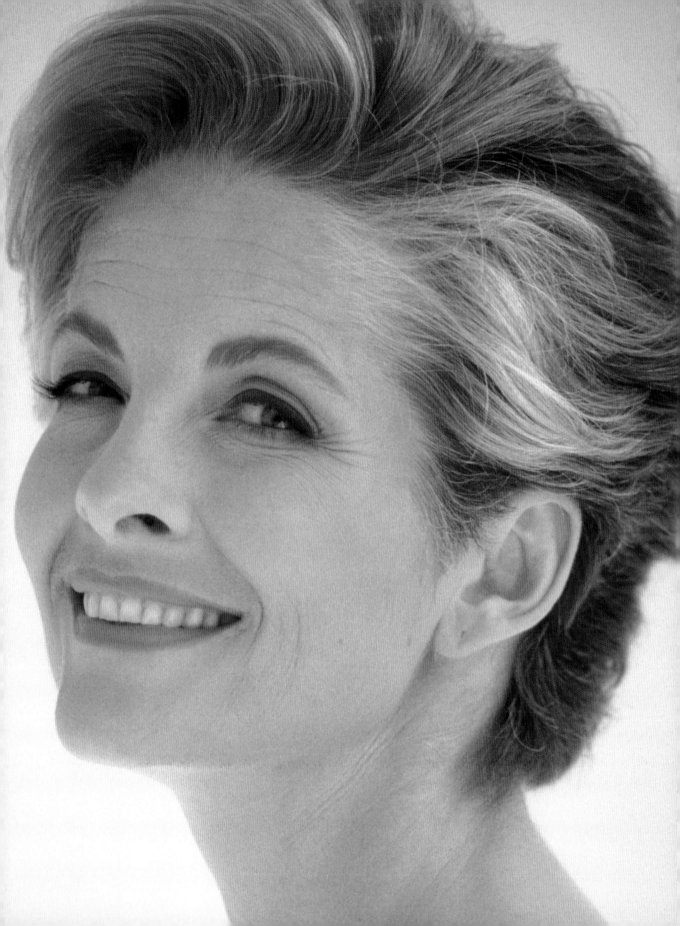

2

HAIR

There are few things more likely to have a strong psychological effect on the way we feel about our looks than the state of our hair.

Having a 'bad hair day' is really a metaphor for having a rotten day all round. If your hair *looks* a mess, you *feel* a mess, and that's the one thing guaranteed to sap a woman's self-confidence. I have absolutely no qualms about venturing out without make-up, but I wouldn't be seen anywhere in public with my hair looking a mess. I often stick it under a hat, or tie it up in a fancy comb; it may not be dressed or glamorous, but it will be tidy and groomed (or out of sight!). That's because I know that scraggy, untidy hair will be a real drain on my confidence. And I'm not alone.

No matter how much care you may have taken over your skin, your make-up or your clothes, if your hair isn't right, you feel a frump.

It's every woman's ambition to have hair that looks healthy and well groomed, regardless of whether you opt for a no-fuss, natural style or, like me, have to use every product and artifice in the book.

Once you hit fifty, even those of you who had trouble-free hair in your youth will find it gets tougher to manage as the colour, texture and density of your hair changes. Mature hair tends to become thin, dry, porous and fragile, so it's essential to adopt the two 'Ms': maintenance and moisturizing. Both have to become a regular part of your anti-ageing regime.

The good news is that it doesn't have to be time consuming, and we don't just have to live with the consequences of mature hair. We can take advantage of every technical, scientific and cosmetic advance to achieve quite remarkable results.

HAIR
Keeping Young and Beautiful

Hair grows by producing brand-new cells below the scalp in hair follicles which are nourished by their own blood supply. When we're born we all have over 100,000 hair follicles, and it's their diameter that dictates the thickness of our hair. Each new cell pushes the one above it to the surface. In young, healthy hair this takes about twenty-eight days. Once the follicles emerge, they immediately die, so the hair we see on our head is in fact a long string of dead cells, called cuticles.

In our mid-thirties the rate of cell production slows down, and by our fifties many of the follicles, in some people perhaps almost half, may have become inactive. So it's taking longer to grow, and we've got less of it.

With the menopause, oestrogen levels start to drop. Oestrogen is food for the new hair cells, so as they're gradually starved of this natural nutrient they start to slim down, getting smaller in diameter. Even if you aren't actually loosing much hair with age, because the individual shafts are thinner, they don't take up as much room on your head, and you start to loose volume.

At about the same time, the melanin pigments, which give each cell its individual colour, start to fade. Once the melanin disappears altogether the new hair cells are produced without colour and the hair becomes grey.

All of these things happen naturally as we mature. Sounds like a real catalogue of disasters doesn't it? And frankly, there's not much we can do to stop them, but what we *can* do is slow the process down and ensure the hair we're left with is healthy and in great condition.

Shampoo

Clean hair is shiny hair, and shiny hair already looks healthy before you do anything else to it. I wash mine every day when I shower in the morning. It's simply not an option to leave it longer than that because I have a tendency towards greasiness so after twenty-four hours my hair rapidly becomes heavy, looks dull and flat, and is impossible to style. The morning ritual of wash, condition, blow-dry and style has become an essential and automatic part of my daily routine. I know that's not an option for everyone, and people with dry hair tend to shy away from daily washing believing it will dry out the hair even more. Not true. In fact, no one should ever go for more than three or, at a push, four days without shampooing. If you have to rely on a weekly visit to, or even from, a hairdresser, take their advice on the best way to maintain your hair between visits.

Hair and scalp tissues are like magnets to dust and grime, especially if you live in a city. A build-up of debris, along with accumulated layers of product like lacquer or styling lotions, will make the hair dull and heavy. Imagine what it would be like if you went for three days without washing your hands. Yuck. So why expose your hair to that level of neglect?

Washing our hair not only removes the grime, but also flattens the rough edges of the individual cuticles. Think of the cuticles as being covered by small scales, not unlike fish scales. A combination of brushing, backcombing, blow-drying, even environmental conditions like the wind and sun, can make the scales stand up, rather like a bird fluffing its feathers. Because mature hair tends to be both fine and dry, it's especially fragile and therefore vulnerable to this fluffing effect. When the scales lie flat against the shaft of the hair, this creates a smooth surface which catches the light, giving the hair a glossy sheen.

You might like to try one of granny's old recipes occasionally – a vinegar rinse. Use 1 part vinegar to 20 parts water. This will remove any final vestige of soap or product build-up, and because the acid in the vinegar will tighten the cuticles, it adds a glossy sheen.

A few companies now produce shampoos especially for mature hair. They contain polymers that help bond the cuticles to the shaft, and so achieve that elusive look we all want as our hair gets older and thinner – the appearance of *volume*.

It's a myth to think you need lots of shampoo producing lots of suds to get really clean hair. A dollop large enough to cover a fifty pence piece is about right for average-length hair. It's more economical, is easier to rinse, and helps reduce the risk of product build-up on the shafts.

Conditioning

It's a mistake to assume you don't need to condition your hair every time you shampoo it, especially if your hair is greasy. Nature intended hair to be covered with a natural water-repellent film to give it sheen, a smooth texture and bounce. No matter how mild your shampoo, some of that film will be washed away so you need to replace it with a conditioner that will help protect your hair from sun and product damage until the next wash.

Don't rub conditioner into your scalp, just disperse it through your hair with your fingers, or use a very wide-toothed comb or brush, so that each shaft gets a coating – but go carefully. Wet hair is fragile at the best of times, so fine, dry mature hair needs a light touch. If your hair is greasy and particularly fine, apply the conditioner to the ends only. Leave for two minutes before rinsing off.

Avoid using a 2-in-1 shampoo and conditioner. They tend to be much too heavy for fine hair and will flatten it rather than giving you extra bounce.

A leave-in conditioner will coat the hair with an extra layer, and give fine hair the appearance of fullness. But again, go easy with it. The whole point of conditioning the hair is to give it body and volume without weighing it down. If you overload fine hair with too much product it will end up looking dull and flat rather than shiny and full.

Intensive Treatment

Every four to six weeks give your hair a real boost with a hot-oil or intensive-moisturizing treatment. Most of the main hair-product manufacturers make them, so you might want to choose one that compliments your usual shampoo and conditioner. Do it when you're taking a long, leisurely lie in the bath. After washing your hair, apply the treatment, then wrap your hair in cling film and cover it with a towel to seal in the heat. Your hair will slurp up the conditioner and feel incredibly soft and manageable afterwards.

Split Ends

Sorry, there is no magic cure. Conditioner will help, but it won't eliminate them. The only solution is to cut them off.

Fine Hair

This is the curse of many mature women, myself included. In fact, I was definitely at the back of the queue when the 'gene fairy' was handing out the goodies in the hair department. Mine is baby fine, dead straight and the bane of my life. If it's not slathered in styling product, then tortured on the heated curling tongs and backcombed into shape, before being smothered in hairspray, it looks more like a bedraggled bird's nest than a crowning glory

Unfortunately, if you have fine hair, but want it always looking well groomed and attractively styled, you're going to have to come to terms with the fact that you have to use a combination of products to create the illusion of fullness. The fact that my hair always *looks* much thicker than it really is, is achieved through a combination of good cut, years of practice and being pretty nifty with a curling tong.

I realize that's not everyone's ideal solution, but these tips should help:

- *Get a really good cut.* Fine hair is easier to manage when it's shorter.
- *Use conditioners and volumizers* – but with a light touch. Too much and the hair will be overloaded and lank, rather than bouncy and manageable.
- Be aware you're going to have to *use more product* than someone blessed with naturally thick or curly hair, and be prepared to take extra care over shampooing out all the residue.
- *Don't rub your hair dry* energetically with a towel. That just encourages the cuticles to rise up rather than stay flat. If you want your hair to dry naturally, blot it with the towel, then gently finger dry by running your hands rapidly through it.
- *If you dry your hair with a blow-dryer, choose the setting that's coolest with the least power.* On the high setting the hair blows all over the place, making it even more fluffy and unmanageable.
- *Turn your head upside down,* and even on the shortest hair, *start from the nape of the neck and work forwards* with the hairdryer nozzle at least 12 centimetres away from your hair. This will reduce the damaging effect of the heat on the cuticles, but at the same time increase the lift at the roots by drying the hair in the opposite direction to its growth.
- If you need to use a volumizing or setting lotion on your hair, top hairdresser Nicky Clarke recommends you, '*Apply products on hair that is almost dry, then continue drying.* That way you use less, and what you do use is more effective.'
- *Use heated rollers or curling tongs* to give extra height, or Velcro rollers with styling spray, and then 'set' by blow-drying.
- *A good old-fashioned hood hairdryer still gives the best results* because it effectively 'bakes' the hair into a new shape around the rollers.
- If you have a casual style, *a hair 'fudge' or structuring cream applied after blow-drying can add extra volume.* Take a very small amount, rub it between your hands to warm it and spread it evenly on your fingers, then briskly run your fingers through the hair. The fudge sticks to the filaments and gives more texture and body to really fine hair.

- On really fine hair, *hairspray is just about essential* to hold the style in place and stop it being blown into a shapeless powder puff. *But don't be tempted to use too much.* The alcohol in the spray will dry the hair even more. I coat my hair in lacquer constantly, especially when I'm filming. It's the only way I can ever get it to stay in place in the teeth of the elements, but I compensate by regularly using shampoos that remove product build-up, and by always conditioning. I find John Frieda's Sheer Blonde especially good. It holds the hair in style without glueing it into a rigid helmet.

Colour

Grey hair can look wonderful on many women and men – especially if it's healthy and shining. But without any help, grey hair has a tendency to go 'off colour' and look dull. To combat this, use shampoos and setting lotions specially formulated for grey or blonde hair. They contain toned pigments that make the hair look clearer. Because grey hair is often coarse as well as fine, the more you moisturize the better it will feel.

Not everyone wants to acknowledge the passage of time by the silver in his or her hair, so a great way to camouflage the effect of gradually greying hair is to include a subtle combination of highlights and lowlights based on the natural colour of your own hair. This needs to be done professionally, and the technician will weave anything up to four

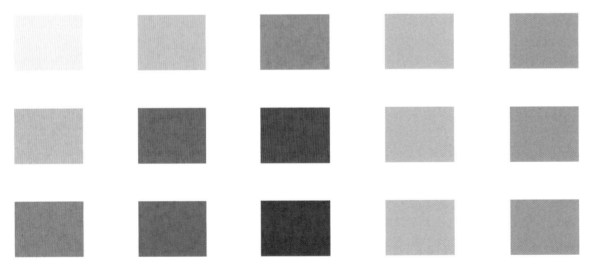

A range of tones and hues will suit your hair as it loses its natural colour, but tints rather than solid overall colour will be most effective and flattering, and easier to maintain.

different colours into your hair, combining lighter highlights with deeper lowlights, what I always refer to as the 'tabby cat' combination. Nobody's hair is exactly the same colour all over, and this streaking effect will disguise the grey, helping it to blend in with the new shades, and give the appearance of volume as the light catches the different hues. It also means you can leave your hair longer between 'touch-ups' on the roots because the regrowth will be less obvious.

If, however, you decide to go for a single colour to hide the grey completely, don't be tempted to try and retain the rich dark colours of your youth. As we get older, classic English skins tend to grow paler, and will look even more washed out if topped by a block of solid, dark colour which is no longer appropriate to your skin colouring.

Keep the same tone, but go a couple of shades lighter and include a few lowlights to add richness and texture and give a more natural look. Lighter shades are much more flattering with age, and a little warmth in the colour helps pale skin look more youthful and healthy.

The disadvantage of an overall colour is that you have to have regular touch-ups if you're very grey because hair grows at approximately a centimetre a month and will soon create a telltale line at the roots.

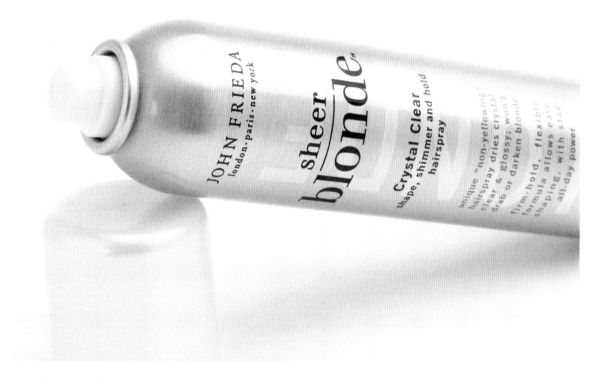

If you have fine hair then you're bound to find you need to use spray for a confident hold, but look around for a product that still leaves it looking natural. Use conditioner regularly, and at least once a month use a shampoo to remove product build-up.

Home Colouring

If colouring your hair at home, remember:

- *Permanent colours are exactly that.* They won't wash out, and are with you until they grow out. Only use products that state on the box that they are specifically for grey hair, because the chemicals are less damaging and the colour will give better coverage.
- *Tone on tone* – usually a gel. They tend to contain low-level hydrogen peroxide to lighten the hair. They gradually wash out, with the effect lasting through twenty or so washes.
- *Semi-permanent colour coats the hair with colour without lightening it.* So grey hair will look highlighted rather than changing colour dramatically. The rest of your hair should gain the appearance of extra texture and body.
- *Temporary colour does what it says on the box.* It gives a temporary shade change, nothing dramatic, which usually washes out after two or three shampoos. Good if you want a quick brightening treatment, or to try out a new shade without long-term consequences.

If you're retouching the roots at home, only apply the lotion to the roots, and not to your whole head of hair. The build-up of colour on hair already coloured not only increases the risk of damage from product overdose, but also distorts the shade you're trying to achieve and you'll end up with a striped effect rather than an overall covering of colour.

Whatever you use, *always* do a strand test. Mature hair, especially grey hair, is *very* porous, so it soaks up colour faster than hair with lots of pigment. You may need to adjust the amount of time you leave the colour on your hair to avoid a nasty shock. You'll only get this right by trying it out first, as I know to my cost!

One Friday evening I slapped on a henna rinse and committed the cardinal sin of *not* doing a patch test. My hair turned bright orange and I spent an agonizing weekend with my head wrapped in scarves waiting for my hairdresser Anthony Mascolo at Toni & Guy to rescue me. They had to strip out all the colour (the henna and my own colour) and then build up layers of brown and blonde to make it look natural. It took over three hours – so I won't be making *that* mistake again.

Naturally Thick or Curly Hair

Oh, lucky you! You probably look at women with thin, straight hair and think, 'What's all the fuss about? We have problems too.' But then conversations with girlfriends over the years have taught me one thing – very few women are ever satisfied with the hair they have.

A good cut is essential for thick hair to reduce some of the bulk and make the most of its weight and natural shape. Next on the list: conditioning. If thick hair gets too dry it has a tendency to matt, making it difficult to brush, and snagging a brush or comb through the hair will damage it and make it even more unruly.

The various anti-frizz and soft-curl serums on the market make a real and immediate difference to thick hair, and straightening tongs aren't just for the twenty-somethings who want to look like Britney Spears or Jennifer Aniston. They're really effective on coarse, mature hair, and could change your style overnight.

You could finish off with a little hair cream or fudge frisked through your hair with warm fingertips to help it to bond together and stop it fluffing up.

Daniel Galvin, one of the country's top stylists, suggests that if you have more than 50 per cent grey in your hair and you're going for an overall colour, you should choose one that is two shades lighter than your natural colour. This adds more texture and movement to the final result. Don't worry if the grey isn't totally covered – solid coverage can look unnatural and artificial

Short versus Long Hair

The great thing about being a twenty-first-century woman is that most of us have enough confidence in ourselves to be able to throw away the rule book that laid down conventions for our mothers and, instead, follow the lead given by fantastic, glamorous role models who are fifty-plus. When it comes to hair length, for instance, there was always the unwritten rule that, 'Long hair is ageing on a woman, hair that's too short and spiky is unflattering, so stick to something simple in the middle.' Then along come Joanna Lumley and Sophia Loren, who both look great with long hair, and Dame Judi Dench, whose feathered gamin cut is as flattering to her face now as it was when she was in her thirties. OK, so we may not all have their collective cheekbones and looks, but clearly the answer is, don't follow convention; follow your own style. Find a length and shape that works for you, and as long as you're comfortable with it, go for it. And don't be afraid of change. If you make a mistake, it will always grow out!

See over for a professional's expert advice on styles that will best suit you.

Anthony Mascolo of Toni & Guy is one of the leading hairdressers in the country. Here are his top six tips for mature hair.

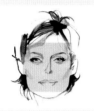

On a square face get the weight of your hair – whatever its length – behind your ears, to soften the jawline.

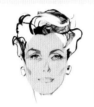

Small faces come alive with hair cut into the nape of the neck.

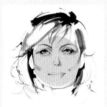

In some women, the face gets rounder with age. Short, spiky hair is rarely flattering to these faces, because it will make them look even fatter. Go for a soft fringe, with layered hair pushed away from the face

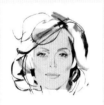

If your face starts to slim down with the years, go for more volume to soften the sharp lines.

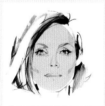

Mature women can look really stylish and sophisticated with a jaw-length bob, but long hair should never lie flat against your head. It will drag down your face, accentuate any lines and look flat and ageing.

Whatever length you choose, to stay looking well groomed aim for healthy, well-conditioned hair that is trimmed regularly.

HAIR
Keeping Healthy

The key to healthy hair is a principle well known to all keen gardeners: feed the roots while it's growing. Once it breaks the surface of the scalp the cells are dead, and therefore inactive. And while there are cosmetic remedies that will improve the look of the hair (see Shampoo and Conditioning, page 36–8) the basic condition and structure of the hair has already been decided during its growth inside the follicle.

Philip Kingsley, one of the country's leading trichologists (hair doctors) reminds us that, 'Hair is protein, and if you add more protein to your diet, especially at breakfast and lunch, this will help feed the hair.'

He suggests you massage your head from time to time. Apart from the fact that it releases tension and generally makes you feel relaxed, the action stimulates the circulation in your scalp and gets more life-giving blood to the follicles.

He also believes that getting the right advice about how to keep your hair and scalp healthy early on in the game will pay dividends as you get older. His philosophy is, 'Don't wait until you've got a problem before seeing a trichologist, make it part of your health routine like visiting the dentist.' Kate Winslett, who's only in her thirties, is already a regular client. But for those of us who've left it a bit late – there are always remedies.

'Whatever the problem,' says Philip, 'we just have to discover the reason, and deal with it.' So menopausal women may need help with their changing hormone levels, while fibroids, for example, will reduce the levels of iron in the system, which can lead to dry, brittle hair. High levels of stress, a poor diet and illness can all affect hair growth, because once the body needs to conserve vital nutrients to cope with these things, the first supply route it cuts is the one to the scalp.

A healthy diet and lifestyle will help keep the scalp nourished, and build a strong foundation for healthier hair.

Perms

For years the 'permanent wave' has been seen as the salvation of every woman who has thin, straight hair. It promises instant curl, body and bounce, and the prospect of being able to manage even the most difficult hair in between visits to a stylist. A good perm can certainly deliver all that, making them an attractive prospect for mature women who see their hair getting thinner, sparser and less manageable with advancing years. The irony is, these are the very women who should be avoiding perms at all costs.

Remember – whatever it may say on the packaging of some hair products – you *cannot* repair badly damaged hair, but you can *protect* it from damage in the first place. That's why regular conditioning and gentle treatment are essential for vulnerable, mature hair.

A perm – even the best of the most modern ones – uses a combination of heat and chemicals to break down the structure of the hair shaft (rather like breaking a bone) and then reset the shaft into a different shape – a curl. Hair that is already thin, with a tendency to dryness, is put under extreme stress by the whole process and will need a lot of aftercare to keep it looking good.

The first rule is: if you can, avoid having a home perm. A professional technician using the latest preparations will assess the state of your hair before embarking on the process and ensure your hair suffers the least possible damage while achieving the best results. If you *do* opt for the home kit, go for something soft. Tight curls that cling to the head like a poodle's are unflattering, old-fashioned and ageing. Working on the back of the head can be especially tricky at the best of times, even more so if your arms or shoulders are a bit stiff. You want to avoid 'kinking' the hair so the curl is uneven, increasing the risk of it breaking, so try to get someone else to help you. It's also easier to get an even distribution of the lotion if you have a friend to help.

But *most importantly*, don't skimp on the 'test curl'. You *must* do a test on fine mature hair. If the chemicals are too strong, or get left on too long, you'll end up with a dry frizz rather than a soft curl.

If that happens, use one of the anti-frizz serums now on the market, and use a rescue conditioning pack to plump up the cuticles. But if the damage is really too bad, then the only solution will be a trip to the hairdressers for a trim!

Once you've had the perm, condition the hair at every opportunity. It won't neutralize the curling effect of the perm, but it will counteract any dryness and help keep the shafts supple, making your artificial curl look more natural and youthful.

One last plea: in spite of the way so many mature women cling to the idea of a perm as the answer to all their hair woes, give it a break. Experiment with some of the styling products and techniques now available that give good long-lasting shape and are far healthier for the hair.

Summer Protection

You wouldn't dream of going out in the sun without some sort of protection on your skin, or at least you shouldn't! (See Sun Damage, page 93.) So apply the same care to your hair.

Sun exposure, especially when combined with salt spray and wind, can play havoc with the general condition of your hair, making it much dryer and also changing the colour. If it's tinted, it will fade more quickly, and highlights can become yellow or brassy. Keep the hair covered whenever possible, with a scarf, baseball cap or a really glamorous straw hat.

If you go swimming and you're going to get your hair wet, cover it in a protective conditioner made specially for swimmers, or use one of the leave-in conditioners which will help protect it in the salt water. Use a shampoo to remove chlorine if you've been in a swimming pool, and don't skimp on the conditioner.

Have a pre-holiday trim to remove any dry, split ends, but postpone any colour treatments until you get back, or a couple of days in the sun will undo all the time and money you spent in the salon.

Wigs

For many women, hair loss and thinning after sixty becomes a real problem. Regular visits to a trichologist can help to slow down the process, but wearing a wig is often the easiest and most practical solution.

For a couple of years in my twenties, I wore a

West End hairdresser and make-over expert Daniel Field tells me the way to avoid split ends is to treat yourself to a silk pillow slip, or cover your pillow with an old silk scarf. At night, tossing and turning on cotton pillow slips means the hair is constantly being 'scuffed', encouraging split ends. But on silk, it slides and avoids damage. It also means you wake in the morning without looking like a rumpled bird's nest. I've tried it, and it works!

succession of wigs and hairpieces to cover up my own offending mop and create the impression of thick, glamorous hair, so I can testify to their practicality, and the feel-good factor they produce on those days when you just can't face the mess that is your own natural hair.

If possible, go for a natural-hair wig, rather than one made of synthetic fibre. The artificial hair always has an unnatural sheen to it, which is a dead giveaway. Try to incorporate some of your own hair around the edges of the wig, especially in the fringe, to conceal the rim and give it a more natural look. Choose a style that looks natural, and not too 'set'. That way you'll get some movement in the hair that will make it look less wig-like.

And remember, many of the great fifty-plus icons like Joan Collins, Barbara Windsor, Shirley Bassey and Tina Turner have been wearing wigs for years, and look amazing.

Choosing a Hairdresser

What is it about a hairdresser that intimidates us so? I've lost count of the number of times in the past I've sat in a hairdresser's chair and watched them slowly massacre or muss up what admittedly isn't much of a head of hair to start with. But I've been too terrified to say, 'That's awful.' Instead, as we view the results of an hour or more of agony with said hairdresser proudly offering a view of the damage from all sides in the back mirror, we smile inanely, say, 'Yes – very nice thank you', and can't wait to escape to the nearest loo to ram on a hat or headscarf and weep over the damage. So new resolution: get a hairdresser you like; a hairdresser you can trust; a hairdresser you can talk to and be honest with. Don't be intimidated, because that's the only way you are ever going to feel really good about your hair and the way you look. My hairdresser for the past ten years has been Anthony Mascola. If he ever retires, or stops cutting my hair, I'm going back to wigs!

One final thought. Whatever you decide to do with your hair, don't let the 'style police' in the media get to you. Styles and techniques that look great on twenty- and thirty-somethings simply don't always work for the mature woman.

I've had a working lifetime of journalists condemning me for my 'dressed' hair. The fact is, I will never feel confident enough to get rid of my heated curling tong, or completely give up the backcombing and the lacquer. They're my security blankets, and I know from experience and years of looking at my face in a mirror and seeing it on television and in photographs, that straight hair, regardless of length and no matter how glossy and well blow-dried, just doesn't suit me.

So if you want to use all manner of products on your hair, have it permed, coloured, hairsprayed or whatever, go ahead and do it if it pleases you. If you defy convention with its length and style, what the heck. As long as your hair remains healthy and in good condition, and *you* are confident with the way it looks, that's all that matters. That way, whenever you face the world you'll look, and feel, a million dollars.

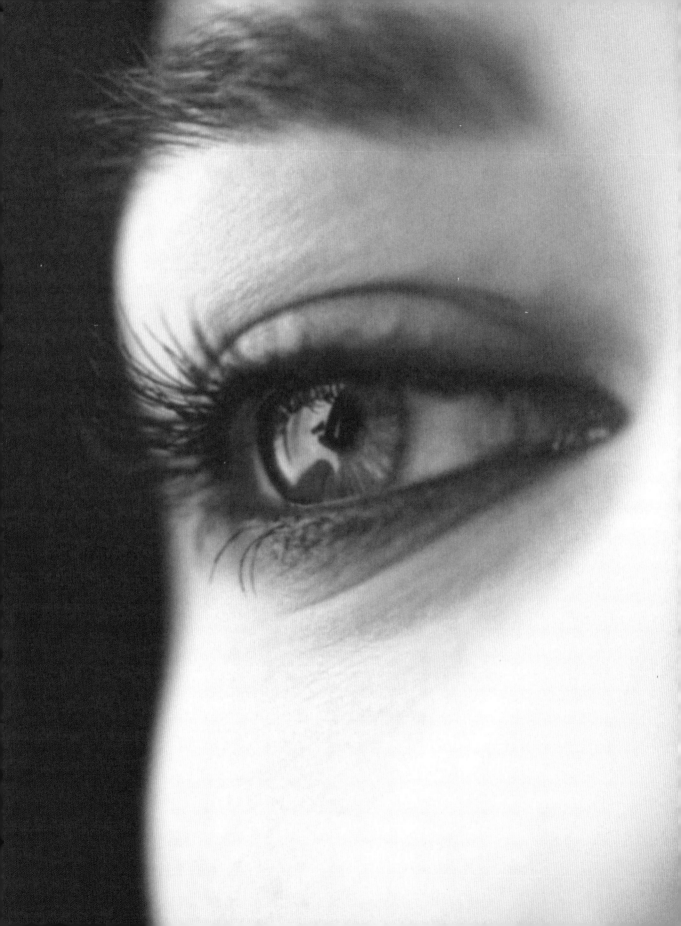

3
EYES

More than any other feature on the face, the eyes have a magnetic quality. We see laughter or sadness in people's eyes; hate, fear, love, tiredness, anxiety, they're all there. No wonder they're referred to as the 'windows on the soul'.

They're also the facial feature we look at more than any other. Just think about it. When we're meeting people, either for the first time or old friends, we tend to make eye contact immediately and then keep returning to the eyes throughout the conversation. They hold our attention and often express what we're really thinking far more eloquently than what comes out of our mouths. But if our eyes are a pretty accurate reflection of our emotions, they're also one of the first areas of our face to start showing the signs of age.

The skin on our eyelids and immediately under the eyes is as fine and delicate as it gets. Loss of collagen and muscle tone contribute to droopy eyelids; squinting against the sun, laughter and a lifetime of animated facial expressions produce crow's feet; poor circulation, rough handling and the general loss of collagen can all affect the under-eye area, producing bags, lines and dark circles.

So if people are going to be drawn to your eyes, let's try and make sure they look as bright, attractive and healthy as possible.

EYES
Keeping Young and Beautiful

For starters, I've always found that one of the best and simplest things we can do to keep our eyes sparkling and healthy is to wear sunglasses. Yes, even in the winter the glare from the sun can be deceptively strong, even through quite dense cloud cover. Overexposure to sunlight can damage the eye itself, while constant squinting against the glare will crease the skin at the corners of the eyes into deep and permanent lines. Sunglasses also have the advantage of covering up a multitude of sins on those days when your eyes would tell the world you're hungover, worn out and feeling anything but bright-eyed and bushy-tailed!

Moisturizing won't get rid of wrinkles, whatever it may say on the packaging. What it will do is plump up the paper-thin skin that lies directly underneath the eyes and make the lines less pronounced. Use a moisturizer specifically produced for the fine skin around the eyes. It won't be quite as heavy as the moisturizer for your face, and will often contain ingredients that will help tighten and smooth the delicate skin. Clarins Beauty Flash Balm is my all-time favourite and Prescriptives Invisible Line Smoother does a great job of 'filling up' the cracks.

Don't overload the eyes with cream. Because the skin is so fine and delicate it can only absorb a small amount. Aim for a drop about the size of a large grain of rice for each eye. Using your ring finger, massage it *lightly* into the skin moving in a circular motion from the outer corner towards the nose and then over the eyelid. Always work towards the nose when handling the superfine skin under the eye, even when putting on foundation. Pulling outwards, away from the nose, will stretch the skin even more. Similarly, if the skin above the eye socket, towards the brow bone, is loose and baggy, you don't want to stretch that any more than is necessary. Use a gentle, but brisk patting action to work the cream into the skin, which should also help improve the muscle tone. Finally, use the ring and middle fingers to lightly and briskly tap the area under the eye above the cheekbone to stimulate circulation. Dark circles under the eyes can often be the result of a sluggish blood supply, so get it moving.

Puffy, tired eyes can be perked up in no time using a teabag. There are powerful antioxidants in tea that reduce swelling, leaving the eyes looking clearer and more awake. Don't use them straight after making your breakfast or afternoon cuppa! The bags need to be cold, so either soak them in cold water before applying to the eyes, or keep a few in the fridge after your morning brew up. Leave them on the eyes for ten minutes and make sure you gently wipe off all the brown stains before applying make-up, or you'll end up with brown, tired-looking smudges and undo all your good work. Alternatively, keep a gel eye pad in the fridge. The ice-cold impact of the mask gets the blood supply rushing to the area to reduce any swelling and is so soothing you can transform your eyes in just a few minutes. Most chemists sell these now and they often come in a form that can also be heated gently to relieve headaches and migraines.

A trick of the trade for tightening up wrinkles around the eyes is to use haemorrhoid cream. You'd be amazed at the number of familiar faces on television who get a dose of haemorrhoid cream under the eyes to make them look less lined and baggy. Just smear the cream under the eye and on the area towards the crow's feet – being really careful not to get it in the eye – and leave it for about four or five minutes. Then wipe off the surplus. Haemorrhoid cream is very gentle and used to shrink piles, and it performs much the same function on fine lines. Always do a patch test on your inner arm to make sure you have no allergic reaction to the cream, and don't use it too often. As an occasional 'quick fix' it's a winner.

The word smoking will crop up throughout the book, accompanied by another single word – don't. Free radicals in cigarette smoke shrink the capillaries of the skin, reducing the blood flow, and affecting the quality and condition of your skin, while the constant screwing up of your eyes against the smoke will give you even more wrinkles. I rest my case!

Cosmetic surgery is the ultimate solution for smoothing out wrinkles, hitching up the droop, removing the bags and giving you younger, wide-awake eyes (see Chapter Nine).

I've had crow's feet (though I prefer to think of them as laughter lines!) since I was in my late twenties. Whenever I laugh or smile the sides of my face crinkle all the way up to my eyes, so the lines are now a permanent feature. But I look at it this way: I've laughed a lot, so the lines are testimony to a reasonably happy life.

Make-up: The Ultimate Camouflage

Eye make-up is designed to enhance eyes and make them look wider, brighter, more awake and less 'aged'. However old you are, a little eye make-up, skilfully applied, can brighten up your face and camouflage many of the signs of ageing that leave you looking tired and washed out. The reverse side of that coin is that too much eye make-up on an older face looks ridiculous and often quite messy because it clogs in the folds and smudges around the wrinkles.

Your watchwords should be 'light and natural'. You want to emphasize the good, camouflage the bad and avoid anything that makes you look like a bug-eyed, sooty-rimmed cartoon.

Start by taking a long, honest look at your eyes and answer these questions:

- Do I have bags and dark rings under my eyes?
- How slack and hooded is the skin on my lids?
- What state are my eyebrows in. Do they frame my face? Are they too thin and too pale?
- Do I have any eyelashes left?

Women friends and magazines may be able to recommend various colours and products that work, but it's only by making an honest assessment of your own eyes that you'll be able to create a make-up 'look' that works for you. My tip? Get yourself a good magnifying mirror. OK, so it will exaggerate imperfections but you'll have a better view of what you're doing, and if you can work either in daylight or a strong artificial light, you'll be less inclined to be heavy handed with the make-up, and get a better, more natural-looking finish when you blend or smudge the colours.

Getting a Good Foundation

Ensure your skin foundation covers the whole eye area. Blend it well in by using your fingertips so it doesn't puddle and sit in the fine lines and loose skin of the lid and under the eye. Remember to work towards the nose, or gently pat and blend the foundation so you don't drag and stretch the skin. Then apply a tiny amount of eye-shadow base or primer to the lid. It will help hold the colour you use, and prevent it from creasing. If you don't use a base, lightly dust loose powder over the lids. But *never* put powder *under* the eye, it will collect in the fine lines and make them look double the size.

Concealer

For dark rings or excessive lines underneath the eyes use either a light-diffusing concealer or creamy stick concealer.

YSL's Touche Eclat is probably the most famous of the light diffusers and works on the principal that tiny particles in the cream will reflect light back from the eye, making it

A light-defuser like Touche Eclat can be worn over make-up to help hide dark rings or excessive lines, but if you want to camouflage you need a concealer like Prescriptives.

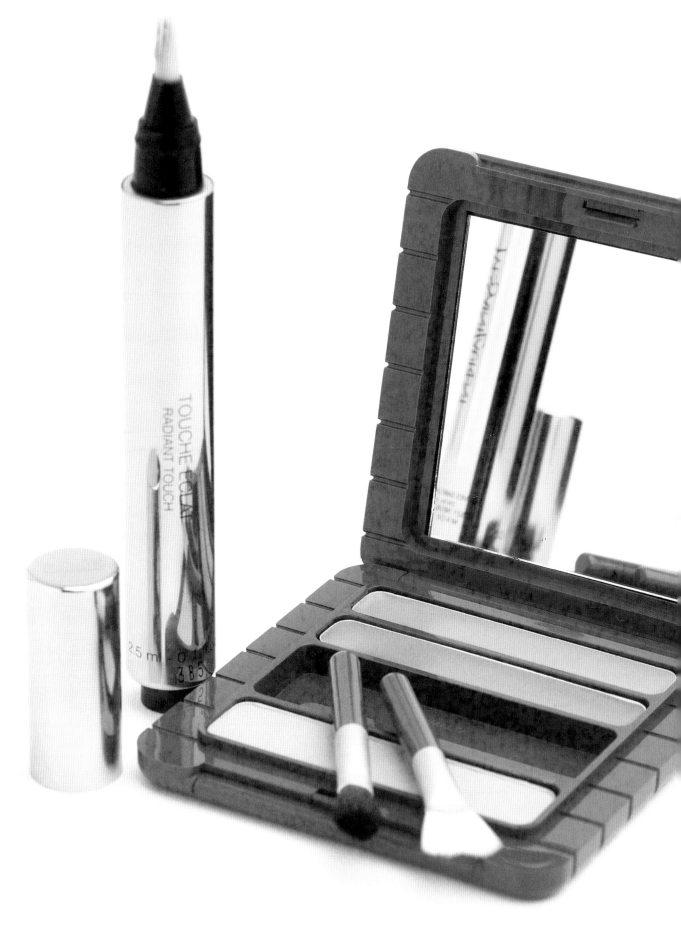

appear less dark and more luminous. It's designed to be used over foundation and usually gives the best results when gently patted into the skin with your ring finger. But there are many other formulas produced by cosmetics houses and you should experiment with them, using testers until you find one with a colour and consistency that's suitable for your skin.

A stick concealer is usually quite thick, and unlike the Touche Eclat is designed to be applied to bare skin *before* your foundation. Avoid those that are too pale, too dry or too greasy. Ideally, they should be creamy in texture and yellow toned. Apply the cream to the area under the eye, making sure you go right into the corner of the nose where you often get a dark smudge on the inside of the nose bone, and gently pat it to blend it in to your skin tone. Don't overload the area, or the cream will clog up the fine lines and make them look more pronounced rather than less obvious.

I find that the light diffuser is fine during the day when I try to have a lighter touch with my make-up, but for evenings I much prefer the coverage of a concealer. The ones by Prescriptives and Kenebo do a great job. On bare skin you can see exactly where the dark lines or imperfections are, block them out and get an even tone to your skin before applying foundation. Whether you're a 'before' or 'after' person, blend the edges into your foundation – you don't want to end up with an obvious set of pale 'goggles' around your eyes.

I'm afraid light diffusers aren't much use on Asian, dark Mediterranean or Afro-Caribbean skins. They are incredibly light in colour and really only work on pale, European skins. People with other skin tones should try using a yellow-toned creamy concealer. It can transform dark circles on black skin when applied before foundation and then blended in with the colour.

Bags are tricky. Draw a fine line of concealer on the lower edge of the bag, to reverse the effect of the shadow and crease, but don't use it on the baggy skin itself. That will only highlight the problem area and make it more obvious. Instead, cover bags with your usual foundation, and smudge a fine line under the lashes to draw the eye away from the puffiness (see Eyeliners, page 56).

If your eyes feel stressed and tired, try one of these pick-me-ups:

Put the heels of your hands into your eye sockets. Block out all the light and apply gentle pressure for about ten seconds.

Get a small 'bean bag' for your eyes. I got one as a stocking filler last Christmas and it's a boon when I want to grab a cat nap. It measures 20 x 10 cm (8 x 4 inches), and is filled with small flax seeds. If you can get a few minutes lying down on the bed or with your head back while you rest in a chair, place the bag over your eyes and relax. The seeds will settle into the eye sockets and the gentle pressure will rest and refresh your eyes.

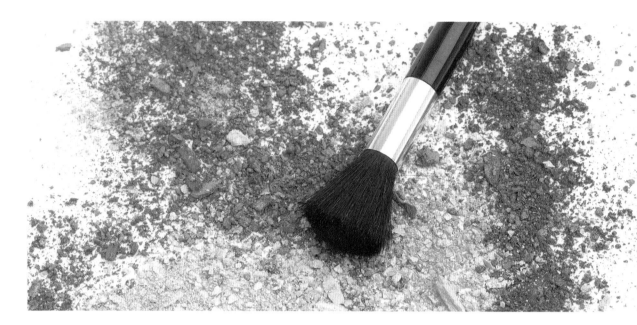

Eyeshadow Colour

This works best on mature eyes when the shades are fairly neutral.

- *As a general rule, go for browns, taupes, dark heathers or greys*, though some mature eyes can take the subtler shades of lavender or pale turquoise. Avoid pinks, rose or any shade that is faintly reddish in tone, as they'll make your eyes look sore and tired.

- Also *avoid bright greens or blues and anything pearlized*, especially if your lids are lined and hooded. They'll draw attention to the lines and exaggerate any imperfections.

- *If your eyes are small or hooded, choose a lighter shade* because darker colours will make the eye recede and look even smaller.

- *Powder tends to be better than cream shadow* because it clings to the surface of the skin for longer, while cream has a tendency to melt and slip into the creases accentuating the lines.

- *Use quite a fat eyeshadow brush* to apply the colour to the lid up to the crease and just onto the bottom of the brow bone and then, *using either using the brush or your fingers, blend*

When applying any powder with a brush give it a good blow, once you've loaded it, to remove the excess. It's particularly important with eyeshadow to reduce the risk of dark powder falling onto your cheeks. Even if you use a sponge applicator, still give it a blow. You'd be amazed at how much powder those little things collect. Remember, girls, we're trying to get *rid* of shadows under the eyes, not create them.

away to nothing so there are no hard edges of colour. If you have a lot of loose skin, by taking the colour slightly above the brow bone you can often disguise the folds of skin and 'lose' them in the colour.

- *Unless your brow bone is firm and line-free, don't be tempted to use a highlighter under the brow.* You're aiming for subtle, not startling, and a highlighter will make the eyes look puffy and emphasize all the camouflage work going on around the lids.
- For evenings, *to create a slightly more dramatic look, try a lighter shade on the lids and a darker shade in the sockets* under the brow bone. Work from the outside towards the nose, and keep the shadow going upwards over the bone. If you bring the darker shade too far down on the outer corners it will only emphasize any droop in your eyelids.

Eyeliners

Eyeliner can open up the eyes and create the illusion of thicker lashes. If you want a really subtle effect, take a fine eye brush, dip it in water and mix a liner out of your powder shadow. It'll produce a slightly darker shade than the lid colour without being too much of a contrast. Personally, I prefer to use a soft eye crayon in either black or brownish black. It's gentle on the skin, and smudges easily into a natural-looking 'shadow' without leaving hard edges.

Whichever you use, start on the top lid at the inner corner, as close to the lashes as you can manage. (This is when you really need a good magnifying mirror.) As you reach the outer edge lift the line slightly and make a small 'V' shape. If you smudge the line with a brush or Q-tip, it will help open up the eyes and make the lashes at the corner of your eyes look thicker.

Under the lower lashes, draw a fine line from the outer corner towards the nose – stopping about halfway along. If you take the line all the way into the corner it can close the eyes up and make them look smaller. Smudge this again, so there are no hard edges. It not only helps give the illusion of thicker lower lashes, it also makes the eyes appear to recede slightly, and draws attention away from any bags or puffiness.

Mascara

Putting mascara on the top lashes will open up your eyes and give them a wide-awake look. I love Almay's Double Lash Mascara, not only because its thickening formula means you only need one coat or because it's hypoallergenic, but also because the wand is really short, so you have much better control over the brush and are less likely to poke yourself in the eye!

Use the best-quality brushes you can afford, and work out a fail-safe range of products for your look.

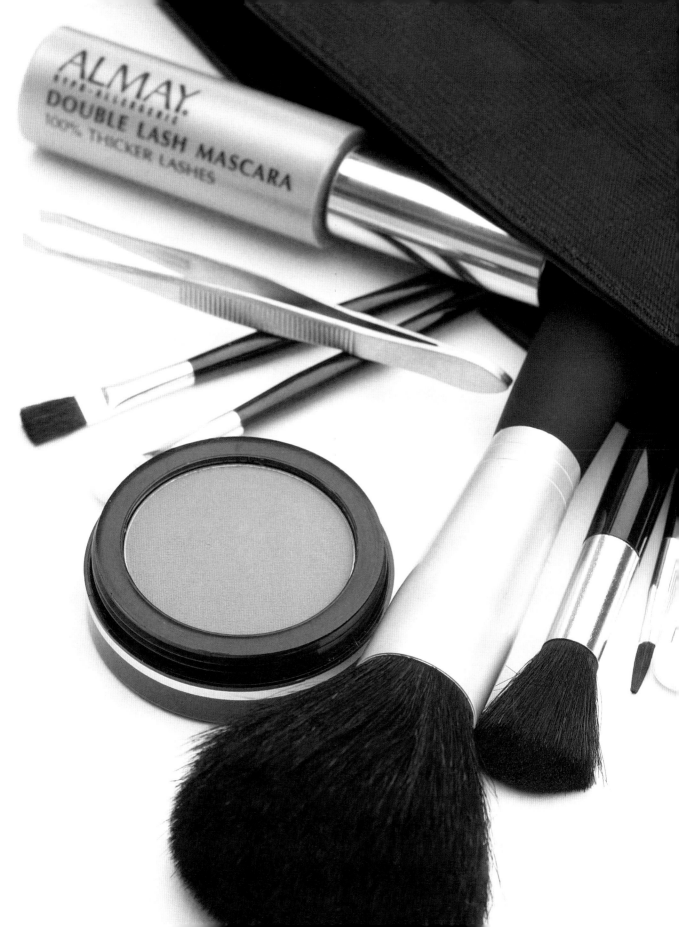

Throw out mascara wands after three months. Any longer than that and they could be harbouring germs which you'll transfer onto your eyes.

Don't overload the lashes, because they'll clog and look really 'doll-like' and messy. A useful tip is to wash an old mascara brush so that it's free of old dry mascara, and then use it to brush the lashes after you've applied the mascara to 'de-clog' them. Don't pump the wand in the cartridge to fill it with mascara, this introduces air into the shaft which will dry out the make-up and shorten its useful life. Roll the brush around the inside of the shaft and pull it out just once.

For the lower lashes, clean the end of the mascara brush on a tissue, and then using just the tip, zigzag the brush over the lashes, or use it to apply the mascara on individual lashes. That way you won't overload them.

If you have very droopy upper eyelids, it's a good idea to use waterproof mascara, which won't smudge onto the skin and make your eyes look sooty.

As much as I love black mascara, it can be too harsh next to some complexions, so go for a dark brown, or as a great alternative – dark navy blue. The slight hint of colour seems to make the whites of the eyes look clearer.

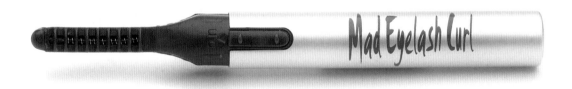

Eyelash Curlers

They may look like mini instruments of torture, but they are a great way of emphasizing your lashes and opening up your eyes, whether or not you wear make-up. My latest 'fab find' is a heated eyelash curler from Mad Cosmetics. The old-fashioned curlers that clamp onto the lashes can, in some hands, be a bit uncomfortable and tricky to use, especially if your lashes are very short. I've discovered the tiny battery-operated wand produces just enough heat in the comb to push the lashes up into a really deep curl, which opens up the eyes miraculously. They're really effective on lashes with or without mascara.

False Eyelashes

These are great fun and a glamorous addition for evenings. Nowadays you don't have to wear the long 'caterpillar' lashes so many of us loved in the sixties. Individual lashes are easy to apply (with a bit of practice and a good magnifying mirror!), and look totally natural when swept with a layer of mascara to blend them into your own lashes.

Removing false lashes should be done after you've used cleanser to take off your eye make-up. The cleanser will help dissolve the glue and you may find the lashes come off on the pads anyway. Don't pull them off harshly, or you could end up pulling out some of your own precious lashes. Bald eyelids – not a pretty sight!

Eyebrows

Eyebrows frame the face and give it balance. As we get older the brows often get thinner and lose colour, but don't be tempted to think that means you have to make them artificially the same shape and colour they were when you were younger. Every part of our colouring, hair, skin and lips, gradually fades with the years, so the colour of our brows should reflect that. Paint them in too dark and they'll dominate your face in a way that can only ever look false.

If your hair is still dark, aim for a brow shade approximately two shades lighter than your hair colour. With blonde-, grey- or ash-coloured hair try a grey or pale taupe. Whatever you choose, the brows should never be a more dominant colour than your hair or they'll look like a heavy mantelpiece rather than a delicate frame. If your brows are particularly light, get them dyed. It's the best way of keeping them looking natural and needing the minimum amount of fuss.

Start by getting the shape right. If you need a bit of help, a trip to a beautician to set the shape is a good idea, and after that you can tweak out the odd hair yourself just to keep them in line.

The American actress/singer/diva Jennifer Lopez (J-Lo) apparently believes her distinctive eyebrows are such an important part of her beautiful image that her 'cosmetics' entourage contains not one, but two eyebrow make-up artists: an 'eyebrow specialist' and an 'eyebrow assistant'.

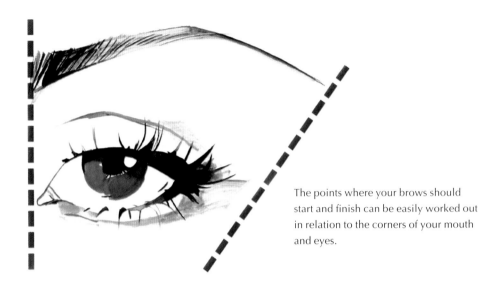

The points where your brows should start and finish can be easily worked out in relation to the corners of your mouth and eyes.

If you are working on them yourself, start by brushing them into their natural shape (I always use a child's toothbrush as I find the head is exactly the right size and texture to do a really good job). Lightly draw in the shape you want, then pluck out any hairs that go beyond that line. Ideally, the brow should start at a point that is level with the inside of your eye. Finding the point at which the brow should end is easy: just lay a pencil or brush on your face and trace a line from the corner of your mouth to the corner of your outer eye. Where the pencil or brush extends beyond that gives you the end point for your brow.

If you are using a pencil to fill in your brows, make sure it's really sharp, and use small, feathery strokes imitating the individual hairs to block in the colour. On mature faces a powder applied with a brush can give a softer, more natural finish. Start with the arch, so you have a point to aim for, then work on the area nearest the nose, and finally the tail of the brow. Don't drop the line too much, as this will appear to drag your face down. Keep everything light, and going upwards. Remember, you want your eyes to look lively and your face looking fresher and more awake.

Brushes

If you're not sure about which shape brushes to use, ask one of the make-up artists at your favourite cosmetics counter. As a general rule, for eyeshadow use a brush with a head that is fat but short; to smudge eyeliners use a narrow, short-haired brush; for eyebrows a narrow, short, wedge-shaped brush. Always go for real hair rather than synthetic, because nylon brushes tend to bend and flick and you could end up with powder speckles on the rest of your face.

Wash brushes regularly – try to do it once a week – using shampoo. It stops the build-up of stale make-up and reduces the risk of infection. It's also much nicer to use clean brushes, and the make-up flows on better.

Removing Eye Make-up

You should do this gently, and *always* before going to bed. We might have been able to get away with forgetting to cleanse in the heady days of our youth – but not any more. Using remover pads, or cotton wool soaked in remover, press the pads onto your eyes for about ten to fifteen seconds. This will give the cleanser time to dissolve the make-up so that you don't have to rub to get it off. You should avoid dragging or stretching the mature skin around the eyes, whenever possible, so giving the lotion time to work means you can be much more gentle and still remove every speck of make-up. Don't forget to swipe along the underside of your lashes where the majority of your mascara is deposited or you'll wake up in the morning with panda eyes!

During my BBC1 newsreading days my eyebrows were always a source of comment. One of my colleague's sons always called me 'Mrs Spock' (after the *Star Trek* character) because of their high arch, while a viewer once wrote accusing me of 'plucking, shaving and torturing' them into shape. For the record – this is the shape I was born with, and it would only be by 'plucking, shaving and torturing' them that I could ever change that!

No Eye Make-up

Many older faces don't need eye make-up at all. Older women whose faces are full of character and life can look vibrant and wonderful without the aid of a whole pallet of artificial aids. What can make a difference is a fine layer of foundation to even out skin tones, tidy brows to give definition to the face, and a sweep of eyelash gel to keep the lashes well conditioned and looking glossy.

EYES
Keeping Healthy

Eyes aren't just a magnetic and attractive feature on our face – they're precious. The trouble is that as we get older, while we might worry about the physical changes to our face and body, and take steps to beat the age clock, we are more phlegmatic about our eyes. We tend to shrug off the fact that we need longer arms to read the paper, or find it difficult to decipher the small print on packaging, and dismiss this as 'one of the signs of old age'. But one of Europe's leading eye surgeons, John Bolger, refuses to be so negative. 'Don't ever say "I'm getting old" and put up with poor vision, because most eye problems associated with old age are detectable, treatable and in the case of cataracts, reversible.'

Cataracts

This is a condition which turns the lenses in our eyes from crystal clear to a milky white. Cataracts disrupt the light entering our eyes and give blurred foggy vision. They are undeniably a symptom of old age, and there's research to show that diabetics are more prone to cataracts, as are heavy drinkers and smokers. There's also a suggestion that trauma and harmful free radicals can promote their growth, so a diet containing antioxidants might reduce the risks. But as John Bolger says, 'No one really knows what actually causes cataracts; why it's possible for an eighty-year-old smoking twenty a day to be unaffected, while a fit sixty-year-old can be

suffering from badly reduced vision. Anyone who can crack that mystery is worthy of a Nobel Prize.'

What we *do* know is that an operation to remove a cataract is one of the few truly successful medical cures that can radically improve the quality of life. The symptoms can be treated, bringing total relief with no need for medication. A winner every time. The operation to remove a cataract is called a phakoemulsifacition. Phako means 'lump' (that's the cataract), which is 'emulsified' during the operation; 99 per cent of cataracts are removed in this way.

A 3 millimetre incision is made at the side of the eye, or under the eyelid, in the white of the eye right next to the iris. If you think of the lens being like a Smartie, then the next bit is easy to understand. A probe first makes a slit in the outer covering of the lens, which is the equivalent of the sugar case of the Smartie. Then, using ultrasound vibrating at between 20,000–40,000 times a second, the milky white of the cataract (the chocolate innards of the Smartie) is broken up and cleaned out, leaving a hollow shell. A new, artificial lens is put inside the shell, and once the probe is removed the shell 'flaps' back into place so there is no need for stitches. The safe removal of the cataract and the ability to liberate the patient from impaired vision is the most important and satisfying function of this operation. But as a bonus, it's now also possible to make the new artificial lens compatible with the glasses you wear, so once the operation is done not only do you get clear vision, but your dependence on glasses can be reduced.

For many years doctors would talk about waiting for the cataract to 'ripen' before removing it. Not any more. Nowadays the operation can be done at any stage in the cataract's growth, at the point when it's bad enough to bother the patient. It's age and size should not be a consideration. So if your doctor trots out this excuse for delaying your cataract operation – don't fall for it. He's ten years out of date.

> When driving, try to wear sunglasses that have Polaroid lenses. They'll cut down the glare from the road and other vehicles, and make driving easier on your eyes.

Weepy Eyes

Every time we blink, there's a whole range of activities going on in and around the eyes. Blinking allows the natural moisture in the eye to be evenly spread over the eyeball to keep it clean and hydrated, while the tiny muscle in the corner of the eye that controls the tear duct is given a squeeze to drain away any unwanted moisture. With age, this muscle, along with so many others in the body, can get tired and less effective, which also increases the possibility of getting an obstruction in the duct. It's when either or both those things happen that you start to get 'weepy eyes' from the build-up of fluid that's not being flushed away,

An obstruction can be cleaned out fairly simply by flushing through the tear duct. But if the muscles fail,

then it's very difficult, if not impossible to rectify. It would involve major surgery to drill through the bone into the nose. It can be done, but it's rarely successful.

Eye Washing

If a foreign body gets lodged in the eye, or if you get a harmful liquid in it, very often the only way to remove it without doing further damage is to use an eye bath or eye drops. But on the whole John Bolger does not recommend the overuse of commercial eye drops. There's a natural antibiotic in our tears that should be sufficient to keep the eyes in good condition. Commercial products can disturb the natural balance in our own formula and reduce our natural defences and immunity to infection. When you have a real medical problem with your eyes, always consult an optician or a doctor. *Don't* try and treat it yourself. Eye infections can sometimes be symptomatic of other problems, so let an expert take a look.

Long hours spent in front of a computer screen (as a silver surfer perhaps!) can produce eyestrain, which can sometimes be eased with eye drops. But what your eyes really need is a rest, and as a treat, a cold compress (see page 51). Similarly, eyes that smart or water in uncomfortable environments, like smoky rooms, don't need washing out – they need rescuing. It's the body's way of saying 'get me out of here' – and that's what you should do.

Glaucoma

This condition occurs when a build-up of pressure within the eyeball becomes so great that it damages the nerve ends carrying images to the brain. Glaucoma can run in families and is one of the most common forms of eye disease in people over sixty. Untreated, it will

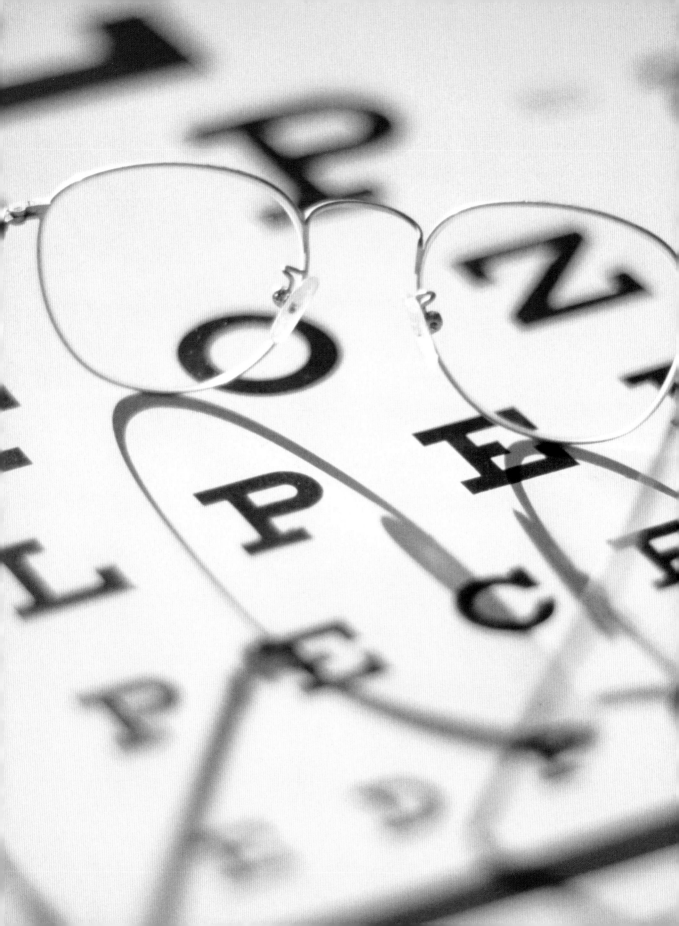

ultimately lead to blindness. The symptoms are so insidious they can go undetected for years, with many people just putting the problem of reduced peripheral vision down to 'old age'. But if you have a regular eye test it will pick up the early signs of the disease, and early detection means it can usually be treated and contained.

Macular Degeneration

By the time we reach seventy or eighty our eyes, like other parts of our bodies, may start showing their age by degenerating and failing to work as efficiently and strongly as they did in our youth. What may start as poor or reduced vision can sometimes progress to a stage where there is a constant black blob in the middle of your line of vision. This is called macular degeneration. It's a bit like what happens when you look into the sun or a bright light, then look away, and find that you have black blobs in your eyes. A regular eye test will pick up early signs, but there's also some evidence that a diet high in zinc and vitamin-packed green vegetables (kale, spinach, etc.) can help to reduce the effects of the disease, and may even prevent its onset. The commercial supplement Viteyes may also help. Tests show that people

taking the supplement had less problems with their eyesight, and the progression of poor vision was slowed down.

Contact Lenses

Many contact-lens wearers find their tolerance to the 'foreign body' in their eyes reduces as their age increases. It won't affect everyone, but if you find the lenses are uncomfortable, listen to your body. It's telling you loud and clear that the 'lens years' are over. So follow the trend set by Madonna, Sophia Loren and Susan Hampshire. Give your eyes a treat, and get some fabulous specs instead.

The most important thing everyone over the age of fifty should do for their eyes is go to an optician once a year for an eye test. Opticians won't just test your vision, they'll also check for signs of disease and be able to detect early signs of diabetes, high blood pressure, cataracts and glaucoma. Getting old does *not* mean having to put up with poor vision.

Regular eye tests are essential to ensure good eye health as much as for practical reasons.

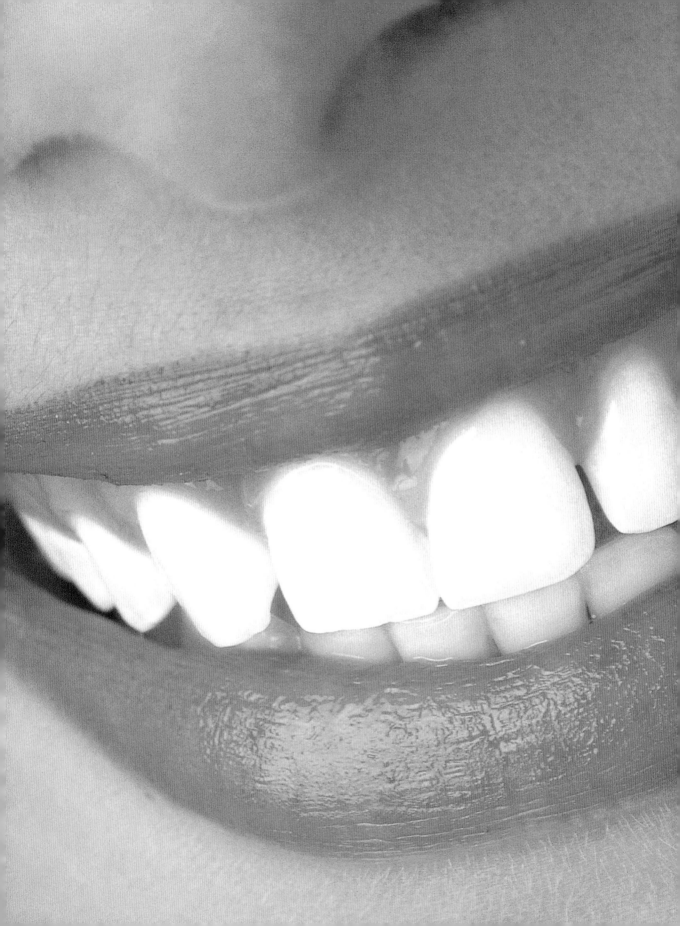

4
LIPS AND TEETH

There is something quintessentially feminine about moist, full lips. As we talk, laugh or smile, people's attention is automatically drawn to our lips and, rightly or wrongly, they make character judgements on what they see: luscious, pouty lips are seen as sexy, while thin pinched lips suggest a mean or sour-tempered person. Neither is necessarily true. The trouble is that the skin on our lips is particularly fragile. It's much thinner and finer than on the rest of our faces (even more so than the very fine skin around the eyes). Lips have no sebaceous glands to keep them naturally supple, so they dry out rapidly from the effects of sun, wind, central heating and other environmental conditions. Perversely, constant licking dries them out more rather than keeping them moist, and as we get older our lips naturally become thinner, dryer and prone to fine wrinkles as they loose their natural deposits of fat. This means the lips are one of our most vulnerable features and therefore, along with the skin around the eyes, one of the first features to display the early signs of ageing. If you're a smoker, all that puckering up around the butt helps form scores of really deep lines on the lips, while the smoke itself releases skin-ageing free radicals that attack the collagen and elastin which are there to keep skin firm and healthy. Clearly, lips need special attention if they're to remain an attractive focal point on our face.

LIPS
Keeping Young and Beautiful

Moisturize

Lips need to be constantly well protected and moisturized. Start the day with a dollop of moisturizer as part of your morning cleanse and moisturizing routine. Work it into the lips, and especially into the skin around the edges to help plump out the fine lines. If you don't wear lipstick, slather on lip balm or lip salves at regular intervals to seal in the moisture and help keep the lips supple. Vaseline is always a good standby, though I'm a huge fan of Liz Earle's Superbalm. A number of cosmetics houses also now make lipgloss in subtle 'barely there' shades so you get just a hint of colour in addition to the gloss and protection.

As lips have no natural defences against the sun, if you're going to be out and about try to use a balm that contains a sunscreen of at least SPF 15. When you see photographs of skiers with their lips covered in white cream, it's not an affectation, but recognition of the damage the pure ultraviolet light in the mountains can wreak on lips. A cloudy day in Britain may not pose such an extreme risk, but the combination of ultraviolet (UV) light and wind at any time of the year will leach all the moisture out of your lips, leaving them parched and dry. So never leave your lips unprotected.

At night, make sure the last thing you do (perhaps after kissing your loved one good night) is lavish on a lip balm. Clarins Age Control Lip and Contour Cream and Elizabeth Arden's Eight Hour Cream Skin Protectant are both wonderful. While you sleep, your lips will have a chance to soak up the moisture without exposure to any of the interruptions posed by eating, drinking and the elements. If you're a smoker and really can't break the habit, then you especially shouldn't skimp on the lip moisturizing regime, and also take lots of antioxidant supplements, like vitamins A, C and E (see Chapter Eleven).

However luxurious or inexpensive your lip moisturizing treatment, make sure you use something!

Elizabeth Arden

CLARINS
PARIS

Baume

Eight Hour
Cream
Skin Protectant
Crème de
Huit Heures
Baume Apaisant
Répar...

LIP THERAPY

Vaseline TRADE MARK ®

PETROLEUM
JELLY

POCKET SIZE

SUPERBALM™

NATURALLY ACTIVE INGREDIENTS

VITAMIN E, ECHINACEA AND PURE OILS OF ROSEHIP
AVOCADO, HAZELNUT, NEROLI, LAVENDER AND CHAMOMILE

30g ℮ 1 oz

Lipstick

Lipstick is a terrific protective barrier. Choose one that has moisturizers in it as opposed to one of the matt types which tend to be much too drying for mature lips. If you have a favourite make or colour that you really don't want to discard, mix a tiny amount of gloss, like the Elizabeth Arden Eight Hour Cream Skin Protectant, into it to up the moisture content. Always keep your lipstick with you during the day, and touch up the colour at regular intervals, especially after eating or drinking, to maintain the protection.

For a great outline and a finish that will last, carry your foundation over your lips, but don't powder – that's too drying. Blot the lips on a tissue. I then like to use a proper lipstick base under the colour because this not only helps to moisturize the lips, it also provides an 'anchor' for the lipstick so it lasts longer and reduces the risk of colour 'bleeding' into the fine lines around the edges of the mouth. Several cosmetics houses make them, but my favourite at the moment is called Liplift and comes from Guerlain.

Next, outline your lips with a lip pencil to give them definition. Use a colour that is one shade darker than your lipstick so the two will blend together, giving your lips shape and definition rather than an obvious border. The waxy consistency of the pencil will also help hold the lipstick in place and stop it bleeding into the fine lines. Choose one that is firm enough to draw a line without flaking, but not so solid that it drags on the delicate skin. I've used Chanel's lip pencils for years. They have the perfect texture, colours that match your natural lip tone, and a built-in lip brush. Sienna is the colour that seems to match most lip colours.

When drawing the line, use short, feathery strokes rather than trying to make one long, continuous line, which can look false and, unless you're very skilled, you're likely to wander off course a bit and get an uneven outline. Take the colour right into the corners of your mouth, so you make a complete circuit of the lips. If you find it difficult to draw on your lips because the skin is too loose or uneven, just part your lips slightly, and draw them back over your teeth. The skin will flatten out and your teeth will form a nice firm base on which to work. On lips that are very thin or uneven, don't start by drawing a 'false' line outside the natural contours of your lips. Follow the genuine line first, and then, if you want to make any part of the upper or lower lip a little fuller, draw a second pencil line on the outside, slightly overlapping the natural line, making the lips a little deeper. Don't be tempted to go onto the skin outside your lips, because if your lipstick wears off during the day it will leave you with a very odd, disconnected line around your mouth.

Lipstick can be as practical as it is beautiful. A base and outlining ensures the look lasts, too.

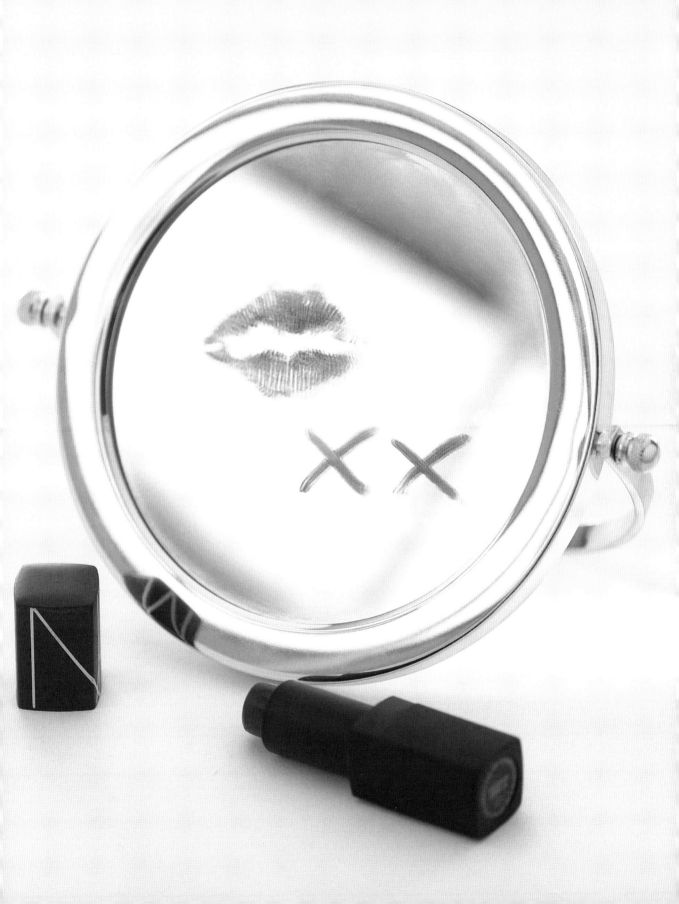

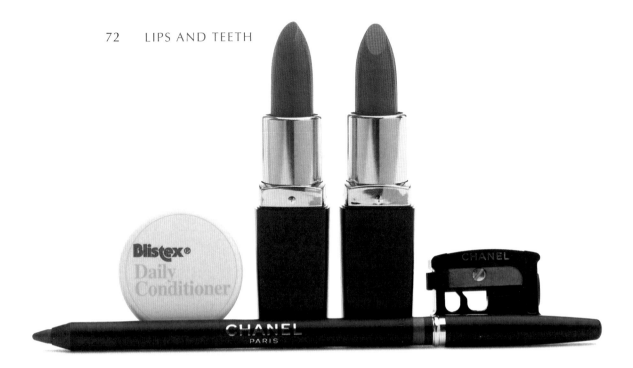

I like to apply the colour with a lip brush; that way I don't use too much, and it's easier to blend into the lip liner. If you prefer to put the lipstick straight on your lips, don't be too heavy handed. You want a film of continuous colour, not a great dollop. The object is to achieve moist, kissable lips, not a great slash of colour in the middle of your face.

Then blot. The great Estée Lauder always said, 'Apply three coats of lip colour. It's the only way to make it last.' It certainly works for me. So, after the first application, blot, put on another layer, blot again, and then finally apply the last coat of colour.

To give your lips an extra plumped-up look, apply a little lipgloss to the centre of the lower lip. But not too much, otherwise the grease will make the colour slide off in no time at all. Or use a lighter shade of lip colour in the centre of the lower lip to give the illusion of fullness.

Finally, to avoid the embarrassment of having lipstick all over your teeth, close your lips over one of your fingers and draw it across from side to side. Any excess colour clinging to the inside of your lips will come off on your finger.

Sore Lips

If your lips do become sore and cracked, apply a coat of Blistex. I keep a tube in my make-up bag at all times. It's terrific for keeping cold sores at bay, works a treat on drying out spots, and is a wonderful salve for sore and damaged lips.

Flaky or Dry Lips

If the skin is flaky and you have loose, dry bits on your lips, don't be tempted to pull the skin off or nibble at them. You'll end up ripping the lip, making it bleed and leaving yourself open to infection. Apply a little moisturizer or balm to the lips, and then gently rub the lips in small circular movements with a damp tissue or fine cloth. The dead bits will gradually flake off without causing damage to the healthy skin underneath.

Lip Enhancement

It is possible to improve the shape and fullness of the lips with a range of cosmetic and surgical enhancements. Collagen or Gortex (yes, the stuff they use to weatherproof your outdoor jackets) can be injected to plump up the lips, or there are gel-like fillers that can give extra volume. The effect lasts from six to nine months, but you must go to a qualified cosmetic surgeon for this work, and don't be over-ambitious with the volume, or you'll end up with the dreaded 'trout pout'. I recently met a girlfriend I hadn't seen for years and almost blurted out, 'What has happened to your mouth?' before I realized she'd been at the collagen. Her lips were so swollen and uneven it looked as though she'd been given a smack in the mouth. Obviously not the look she'd intended.

Lip grafts are easier to control, and a permanent solution to thin lips. The surgeon will graft a small piece of skin and fat cells, usually from your abdomen or buttocks, into the lips giving them a natural, soft fullness that will last for ever (see Chapter Nine).

But if none of that appeals, just smile. Seriously. Smiling not only brightens up your whole face, it also flattens out the lines around your lips, and exercises the very muscles that help keep the lips and mouth firm. Also, while no one's looking, you could try this simple exercise a couple of times a day. Just say 'ee, oo, ee, oo' several times over to really work the jaw and lips. Every little helps.

TEETH
Keeping Healthy

If your lips are in great shape, and you've got a terrific smile, the last thing you want to do is spoil the effect with a mouthful of poor teeth.

I remember as a child, that both my parents already had a couple of false teeth when they were in their thirties. In fact, up until the 1960s it was quite common for reasonably young and middle-aged people to find themselves with a mouthful of dentures. Improved dental techniques and fluoride have thankfully made all the difference in the world, so that nowadays false teeth are the exception rather than the rule, and we all have the opportunity of holding on to most of our original teeth for a lifetime. But we have to recognize that gums in particular change radically with age, and maintaining good teeth into your eighties and beyond will take a little more effort than just brushing twice daily.

With a bit of luck, and regular attention, you should be able to hang on to the pearlies, pain free and trouble free, for a few more years.

Dental Treatment

Book an appointment with your dentist or hygienist every six months to keep on top of good dental health. If you've got out of the habit because you're unhappy with your current dentist or, like many people, have a genuine fear of sitting in that chair and exposing yourself to the horrors of high-tech machinery and possible pain, ask around and see how other people fare. Often the best way of finding a really good dentist is by talking to friends who can genuinely recommend their own practice. If you want an NHS dentist as opposed to a private practice, ring NHS Direct for the name of your nearest surgery.

Home Dental Care

A regular maintenance routine at home has the biggest impact on dental health. Brushing every morning and evening is a must, preferably with a toothpaste containing fluoride for maximum protection. With age, the enamel on our teeth can start to thin, making the teeth more porous and therefore sensitive to hot or cold food and drinks. If that happens, switch to a toothpaste made specially for sensitive teeth like Sensodine, which will leave a protective film on the enamel and cut down the pain level. Or ask your dentist to coat your teeth with a product called a fluoride varnish. I have this done every six months and it helps enormously.

Take a close look at your toothbrush. If the bristles are too harsh they can irritate and even damage the gums, which do become more sensitive with age. And don't get too attached to the brush. If you use a soft bristle, after four to six weeks it's out! A medium-bristle toothbrush might last for two months, but no longer. Beyond that, the bristles become too distorted and less effective in cleaning between the teeth, and they'll be harbouring all sorts of bacteria you don't want to put back into your nice clean mouth.

Flossing

Flossing must become an essential part of your daily dental-health routine. And this is why: as we get older, our gums naturally recede (hence, 'long in the tooth'). This not only exposes the lower part of our teeth, nearer the roots, it also widens the gaps between our teeth where food and debris can lodge. It only takes a small amount of debris to promote the build-up of plaque (that nasty, yellow, cement-like stuff that forms at the bottom of our teeth) and encourage bacteria which attack both the tooth enamel and the gums, leading to gum disease and root decay. Nowadays, gum disease causes more teeth to be lost than tooth decay, it can also be a cause of bad breath.

So, take a look in the mirror. If you can see the build-up of plaque, or if you're spitting pink-coloured toothpaste into the sink in the morning because your gums bleed when you brush, then you know you've got problems.

When we're young we produce a lot of saliva which is chock full of natural antibacterial ingredients, but with advancing years, our saliva output decreases. It can also be affected by some medication, like blood pressure or heart pills. So our natural defences are gradually reduced and made less effective with age. Many people also acquire a sweet tooth and the sugar from chocolates and sticky toffees just loves to cling to the teeth, slowly but surely turning into acids which eat into the enamel. That's where the flossing comes in. Done regularly, especially at night, it will clear out

any particles that may be lurking between the teeth or on the gums and reduce the risk of infection.

A useful tip: cut off a piece of floss about 25 centimetres long and tie it into a loop. It will be easier to hold, and you can use a clean section of the floss every time as you work your way around your mouth between the teeth. Alternatively, buy what my dentist calls a 'Christmas tree' brush. It's a tiny V-shaped brush (a bit like a Christmas tree!) which you gently poke between your teeth to give your gums a really good clean.

Follow with a quick swill of mouthwash to zap any bacteria still clinging to the gums, and you can go to sleep safe in the knowledge that there aren't armies of germs attacking your teeth and gums during the night.

Yellowing Teeth

As we get older our teeth produce more of the yellowy-brown dentine inside the teeth, while the bluish-white enamel gets thinner. The result? Teeth start to discolour and look more yellow with age. Regular visits to the hygienist can help keep the teeth white and healthy.

Teeth Whitening

Ageing apart, years of smoking, drinking red wine or eating foods likely to stain your teeth can leave them looking dull and discoloured. Until recently it was possible for dentists to apply a substance that would clean up your teeth and return them to a healthy, sparkling white. However, current EU legislation on this subject is being interpreted by the Department of Trade and Industry in a way that makes the use of this substance in Britain illegal, even though paradoxically it can still be used in the USA and other parts of

Europe. According to the British Dental Association, 'Whitening is one of the safest and least invasive treatments we can offer.' So consult your dentist; he or she may have a solution and given time, the legislation should be clarified.

If you'd like to try the DIY approach, Boots make a home-whitening kit which is simple and safe to use and could make all the difference to your smile in no time.

Cold Sores

Cold Sores are painful and unsightly, but if you catch them quickly enough you can prevent them from forming into large crusty sores.

They are the result of the herpes virus, which most of us carry in our systems. Most of the time they stay dormant, but they can be triggered into action by stress, fatigue, illness (like a cold or flu) and sunlight. The first hint you're about to get a break out is a tingling or itching sensation on your lip. My tip – grab a bottle of tea tree oil or a tube of Blistex. Keep dabbing the spot with the cream or oil every hour or so. The sore will run its course, but if you can keep up the treatment, I usually find that it never manages to form a crusty, bloody scab. Instead, you get a bit of a sore lump that can be easily concealed with make-up, and goes within a day or two.

Ignore both flossing and cleaning your teeth at your peril. Reinforce your home regime with hygenist visits, and ask about the latest information on whitening procedures.

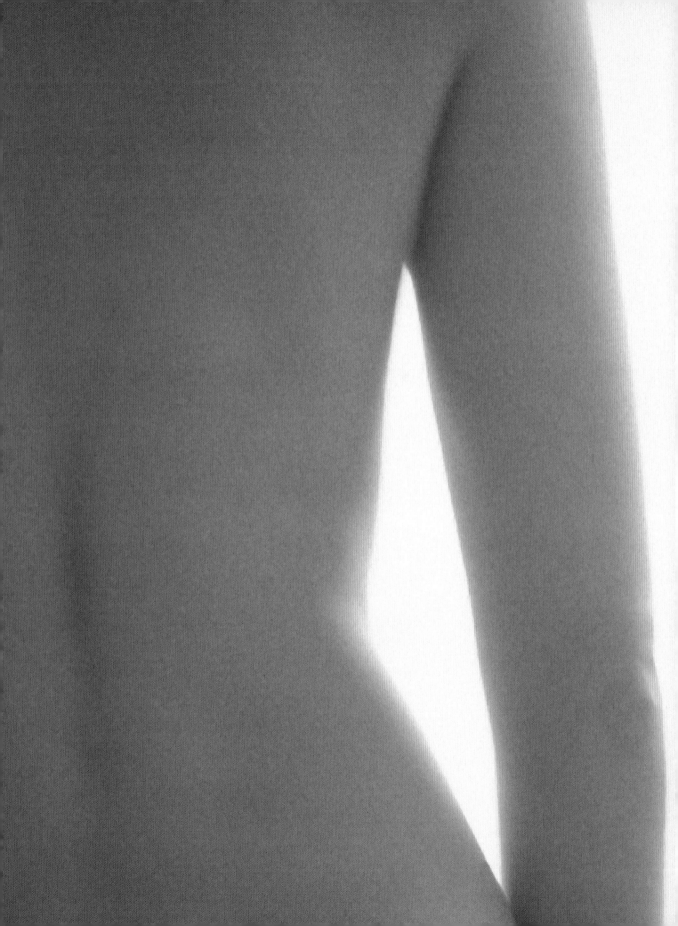

5
BODY MATTERS

It's unlikely that many of us have ever had the 'perfect body'. Throughout life it seems there have always been bits we love and bits we loathe, bits we want to improve, are proud to expose or would rather keep under wraps. So it's quite nice to hit middle age and realize that with maturity comes the wisdom to be more comfortable with what we've got and who we are, and to recognize that being fit and healthy is more important than being cover-girl thin, and knowing that if there *are* areas we want to work on, we'll be doing it for ourselves and not the universal approval of the 'fashion police'.

Most of us have to accept that our hips will get a bit wider and our tummies a little rounder. Hormonal and lifestyle changes mean that excess fat in the body makes a beeline for those areas in middle age. But then women are supposed to have curves, so providing you can keep your body active and fit, is it really such a big deal if you no longer have a washboard stomach? We can all take heart from a recent survey that showed 52 per cent of men prefer their women to be voluptuous with a few womanly curves. But while recognizing that age and gravity are going to rob our skin of elasticity and tone leading to the inevitable wrinkles, what we *don't* have to do is let them take over and leave us looking like an old prune.

OK, so I can no longer fit into my wedding dress. At twenty-four, I weighed 47 kilos (7st 6lb) and was a tiny size 10. Thirty-plus years later I'm 12 kilos (2st) heavier and a comfortable size 12, and there are lumpy bits and wrinkles I'm never going to shift. But I still have bags of energy, supple joints and skin that doesn't resemble the Dead Sea scrolls. I look after my body. I know its strengths and limitations in supporting the active lifestyle I lead. I'm good to it, and in return I feel fit, healthy and confident that my body will go on allowing me to enjoy a full and active life and to get on with the things I really enjoy. So let's get to work on a few body matters.

BODY MATTERS
Keeping Young and Beautiful

Skin

Our skin is the largest organ in our body and performs a whole series of amazing functions. It protects us from the elements, and from all manner of environmental damage, dirt and temperature change. It maintains body temperature, regulates body fluids and acts like a massive waste-disposal unit by getting rid of toxins and rubbish throughout the day.

The general condition of your skin will be affected by age as you naturally reduce collagen production and by poor diet, smoking, excess alcohol, illness, some prescription drugs, lack of exercise and overexposure to the sun.

Keeping skin healthy and supple means giving it help from both inside and out. You can do this by feeding it and keeping it hydrated while the new skin cells are being formed down in the dermis, and by exfoliating and moisturizing once the cells reach the surface.

Food and Drink

Try to ensure you eat plenty of fresh fruit and vegetables each day to give you a natural intake of minerals and vitamins. Vitamins A, B and C are all essential for healthy skin. Topping up with mineral and vitamin supplements from the health food shop is never a bad thing. But don't overdo it. Take only the recommended daily dose and check with your doctor that the supplements won't react with any other medication you might be taking.

One of the most important things you can do for your skin is to keep it well hydrated by drinking at least 1.5 litres of pure still water during the day (coffee and tea don't count because their caffeine content is dehydrating).

Even though we may think our bodies are pretty solid with all that flesh and bone holding us together, in fact we're made

If you'd rather not drink bottled water, buy a water-filter jug to filter tap water and keep it in the fridge. In some parts of the country the tap water is wonderfully pure and sweet. But in others you're better off with a filter!

Don't wait to feel thirsty before you drink water. The benefits of drinking at least 1.5 litres a day can't be over-emphasized.

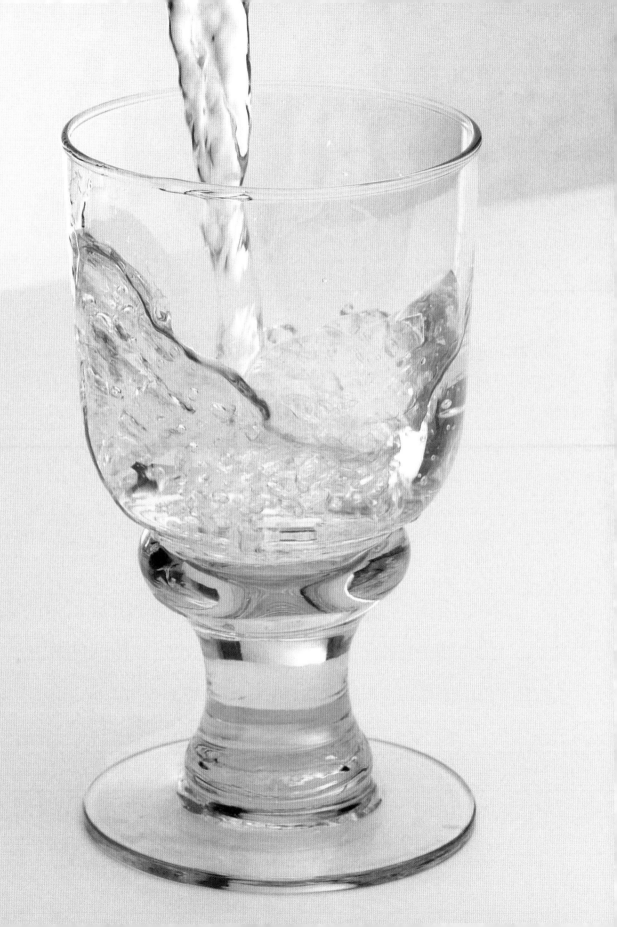

When you should drink more water
- *On a plane journey*. Low humidity means you should drink at least a full 250ml glass of water for every hour in the air.
- *In hot conditions* when you perspire more, *and in cold conditions* when water evaporates more quickly from your lungs *as you breathe*.
- *Smoking* can be dehydrating. Smokers should ensure they always drink at least 1.5 litres half a day, and preferably 2 litres, to compensate for the extra dehydration.
- *Caffeine and alcohol* dehydrate the system. Drink a glass of water for every caffeinated or alcoholic drink you consume.
- *When you're ill*. Water will flush out the system and help prevent the dehydrating effect of some medications.

up of approximately 70 per cent water. Most adults lose about half a litre of water every day through perspiration and breathing, and if you're exercising you loose a lot more. It all has to be replaced to flush out toxins, keep our kidneys in good condition, move nutrients around the body and maintain hydration levels. Think of an apple left standing in a fruit bowl for a couple of weeks. As the moisture in the flesh dries out, the skin shrinks and wrinkles. That's what happens to your body if you don't keep its water reservoir topped up.

Some research done recently in America suggests water helps keep you slim and trim as it flushes out excess waste products. It certainly helps prevent water retention, which usually occurs when the body thinks it's going to have its water supply switched off, and goes into panic mode and starts storing water.

Feeling thirsty is the body's way of telling you it's already dehydrated, so don't wait for that to happen. Drink water regularly throughout the day. As our brains consist of about 75 per cent water, even a small reduction in hydration can affect us, leading to headaches and an overall feeling of sluggishness.

Ever since I had food poisoning in the late eighties, I've been unable to drink milk, so I drink water and herb teas instead. I start every day with a mug of hot water (sometimes with a slice of lemon) and just keep drinking the stuff throughout the day. I get a few funny looks from people who can't believe that's really all I want, but I rarely, if ever, get headaches, and my skin stays in pretty good nick.

One of the best ways to check on whether or not your body is dehydrated is to keep an eye on the colour of your urine. Ideally it should be quite pale in colour. If it's dark, you're not drinking enough.

You can also try the 'pinch' test. Pinch the skin on the back of your hand or your forearm near the wrist. If it springs back nice and flat your skin is well hydrated. But if it sits there in a ridge and oh so slowly flattens out, grab the water bottle – your skin is parched and desperate for moisture.

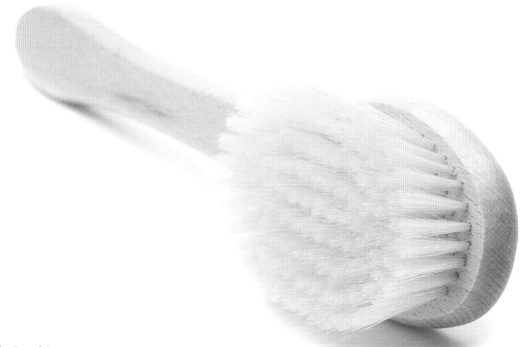

Body Brushing

This is one of the simplest, most effective things you can do to improve the quality of your skin. Brushing, using a natural-fibre body brush, will sweep away dead skin cells, aid circulation and stimulate the flow of lymph – the milky fluid in the body which plays an important part in maintaining the immune system and clears out toxins and waste from the body.

Always brush on dry skin. If it's damp, it could stretch, and that's the last thing we want on mature skin!

Use long, firm strokes, starting at the ankles and working your way up over the legs, knees, thighs, tum, hips and bum. Begin with fairly light strokes, but as you get more used to the sensation you can increase the pressure on the brush. *Never* brush sore, ulcerated skin or over varicose veins.

Brush gently around the waistline and over the tummy, then across the shoulders and down the arms, paying particular attention to the insides of the arms from the elbows to the armpits. Always brush towards the heart in the direction of the blood flow.

This can really help reduce puffy ankles through increased circulation, and will eventually work wonders on fatty deposits like cellulite. It's not an overnight miracle cure, but the brushing helps to break down the hard deposits of fat that are lurking in the cells, giving your skin that orange-peel look, while the stimulated lymph flushes the waste out of your system (see Cellulite, pages 112–5).

Moisturize

Our skin is constantly renewing itself over a twenty-eight-day cycle. That's roughly how long it takes for the brand-new cells being created down in the dermis to reach the surface. While they're being formed they're getting plenty of protein and water from the body. But as they work their way up through the 'sandwich' of dermis, epidermis and stratum corneum, they're cut off from their natural food supply and gradually die. This means that by the time they're exposed to the outside world they're already dead and consist mainly of keratin, the tough fibrous protein also found in hair and nails.

So they just sit there, flat and dead, forming the outer layer of our skin. Think about it. The cells have gone for weeks without water. They're parched and thirsty, desperate for a drink (well, wouldn't you be?). That's why we need to start hydrating the skin from the outside.

Exfoliating the body is just as important as exfoliation on the face, and is an important part of maximizing the effect of moisturizing lotions. How often have you run your fingernails over your skin while lying in the bath and collected a grey gunge under your nails. It's not dirt – it's dead skin cells. That's what you need to remove with a salt scrub or body exfoliator. The mild scrubbing action will stimulate your circulation and reveal younger, fresher skin underneath.

When you emerge from a bath or shower, don't be tempted to towel yourself absolutely dry. You should certainly dry between your toes to prevent fungal infection, and in any other nooks and crannies. But leaving your skin slightly damp will give the cells a better chance to absorb the moisture. So apply your body moisturizer straight onto damp skin.

All moisturizers contain water and a form of lubricant. The water will be absorbed by the dry skin cells, and then sealed in place by the oils and creams, which in turn will soften and lubricate the surface.

Always pay particular attention to elbows, knees and shins. They have less sebaceous glands than the rest of the body, so they don't produce much of their own natural lubricant. Add this to the fact that collagen production is severely depleted with age, and you can see why we get such wrinkly elbows, saggy knees and dry shins as the birthdays roll round.

Be lavish with the cream, rub it in well and make it an opportunity to give yourself a bit of a massage while you're doing it. Use your thumbs to ease any stiffness in your leg

An exfoliating scrub will aid in the skin-renewal process, and prepare the skin to receive a moisturizing treatment.

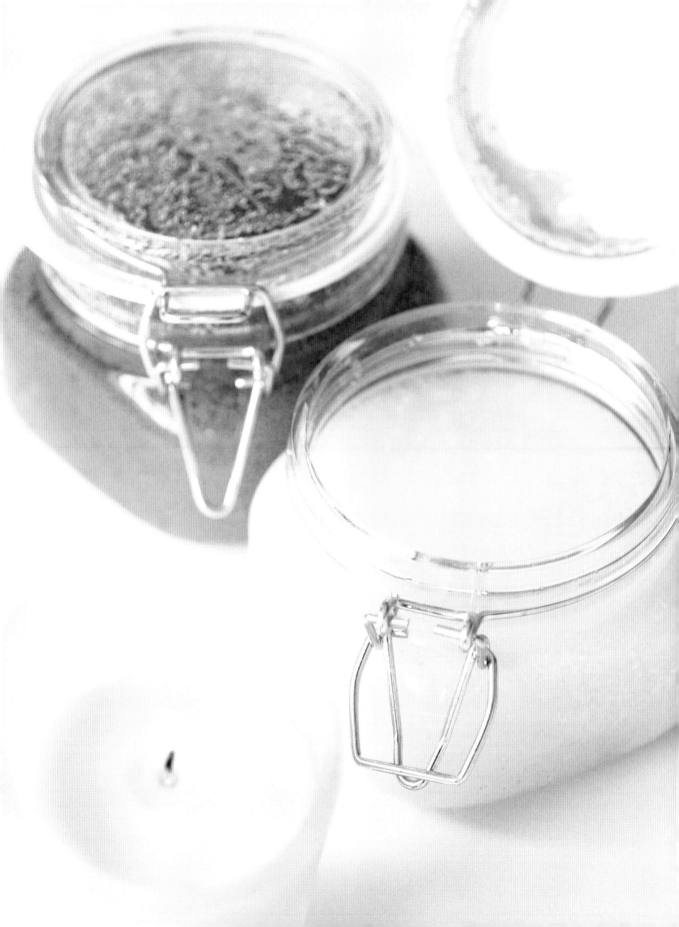

muscles and work them into the muscles of the upper arms to help keep them firm and combat sagging flesh. Let your fingers dig deep into the muscles on either side of your neck, across your shoulders and into the main lumbar muscles in your back. It's also a good time to do a regular check for lumps in the breasts. As you smooth on the cream you can immediately feel any irregularity (see Cancer, page 162).

Fake Tans

There's nothing like a bit of healthy sun exposure to give us a lovely glow, fill us with vitamin D to help our bodies absorb calcium and make us feel generally good about ourselves. Sunlight really is essential to human beings. But just thirty minutes exposure a day gives you all the exposure to vitamin D you need. More than that, on badly protected skin, and you're storing up real trouble for yourself (see Sun Damage, page 93).

A fake tan will not only give you a great colour, year round, it's also healthier for you, and currently the fashionable thing to do.

Beauty salons offer all manner of treatments, ranging from the straightforward application of a fake-tan cream via massage, to the latest technology which lets you stand in a cabinet and get blasted by a fine spray of fake tan which covers your entire body in a matter of seconds. The result is a glorious, all-over light tan, which can be intensified in colour by repeated applications.

Nowadays, fake tans are so easy to use you can often achieve a perfect colour at home, without risking the awful orange streaks that were a feature of the 'fake' look some years ago. They work especially well on legs, which are always stubborn to tan in natural sunlight. I've found that Decléor, Lancaster, Clarins and Saint Tropez make some of the best home kits, but ask friends and see how they've got on with the various makes on the market. Personal recommendation is often the best way to start if you haven't tried these creams before.

For a perfect finish just follow these simple rules:
- Always begin by exfoliating the area you're going to treat. Fake tans only last for about three weeks at the most because dead skin cells are shed, so you want to start with the freshest, newest skin possible. Exfoliating will also give you a nice smooth surface on which to apply the cream.
- Next, moisturize. The cream will hydrate the skin, making it more responsive to the colour of the fake-tan product.
- Leave the skin to rest for ten minutes or so, then apply the fake-tan cream with long, even strokes. To avoid a tide mark on your feet, gently wipe the area with a damp

cloth to even out the spread of the cream, especially around the ankles and toes. Do the same on your knees and elbows, which on mature skin can be drier and more creased, so they tend to hold the colour and leave you with blotchy patches.

Fake tans for the face usually produce a lighter shade, and give a wonderfully healthy glow. But don't overdo them, or you can end up looking like an orange on a stick. For a gentler colour try one of the after-sun creams that contain what are called 'tan prolongers'. All the major sun-cream manufacturers now produce them, and they're just lovely moisturizers with a small amount of fake tan included. The result is a well-moisturized skin with just a hint of natural-looking, sun-kissed colour.

Take a Bath

As someone who likes to start the day with an invigorating shower, lying in the bath is something I only do as a real treat when I want to switch off completely and have a long, relaxing soak. There's a lot of research around to show that soaking in the bath is not just an indulgence. It really does help the body to de-stress and shed toxins and has a therapeutic effect on both the mind and body.

We all know the beneficial effect of relaxing bath oils and warm water on easing the pain and tension out of muscles after a hard day's work. While simply lying in the bath letting the water take 90 per cent of your weight reduces the stress on joints and muscles. But sometimes it's just your mind that needs relaxing, in which case a few drops of essential oil like geranium or lavender added to warm water help produce a feeling of well-being and total relaxation.

Natural health guru Liz Earle swears by Epsom salts. She says adding a kilo to the bath water will really ease out tensions and help the water soak out toxins and waste that might be clogging up the skin cells. I know a kilo sounds a lot, but that's how much Liz says you need in the water to really get the benefit.

If you have the time to indulge yourself, put on a face mask and pop a couple of iced cucumber slices or cold teabags on your eyes to reduce puffiness (keep the teabags from your last couple of cups of tea, pop them in the fridge so they're nice and chilled, and wring them out in cold water before applying).

You could even give yourself a body scrub to exfoliate the topmost layer of dead skin cells. Origins make a fabulous salt rub. Make your own by applying a handful of household salt to a sponge or flannel, mixed with soap or bath lotion. Pay particular attention to heels, elbows, shins and knees where the skin becomes particularly dry and scaly. Believe me, your skin will feel like silk afterwards.

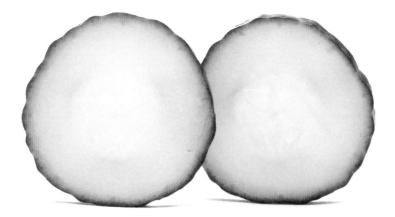

If you shave your legs or bikini line, just before you get out of the bath is a perfect time to get a really close shave. Coarse hair – like that on the legs – needs at least five minutes soaking in water to become soft and pliable, and therefore easier to shave.

A final thought – for pure indulgence, lower the lights in the bathroom, or replace them altogether with candles. Hedonistic *and* romantic!

Massage

Don't ever underestimate the power of human touch. There's something so very comforting about being given a hug or just a squeeze of the hand in moments of stress or emotional pain. Whenever any member of your family falls over and hurts themself,

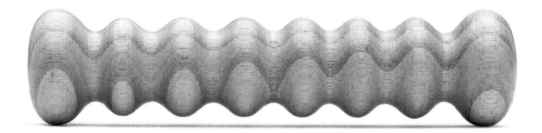

how often have you caught yourself saying, 'Let me rub it better'? The mere act of rubbing the skin releases extra endorphins, the body's natural painkillers, to ease the hurt and speed up recovery. That's why massage is such a wonderful way of easing stress and muscular pain and produces a feeling of general wellbeing, and also why it's being used increasingly in hospitals and hospices, especially hand and foot massage, to bring comfort to patients.

Depending on which style of massage you choose, if you quite literally put your body in the hands of an expert you can be invigorated to beat lethargy and deep-seated aches and pains, or soothed into combating headaches, stress and insomnia. In some cases massage can even help digestive disorders and problems with circulation.

Swedish Massage

This is the most commonly recognized style of massage in Europe. It combines light stroking of the muscles with long, firmer strokes and a gentle kneading to relax the body. It releases toxins, improves circulation and eases aches and pains. A good masseur will always ask if you want a 'deep' or a 'gentle' massage. Only you can decide on the level of pressure your body can stand, but the firmer the stroke, the more effective the treatment.

Aromatherapy

This is massage using essential aromatic oils and is especially valuable in releasing emotional tensions. The oils are too concentrated to be used neat on the skin and should always be combined with a neutral massage oil.

- *Lavender* is wonderful in helping you relax. Lavender pillows or a few drops of essential oil on your pillow can help you sleep. I keep a spray of lavender water next

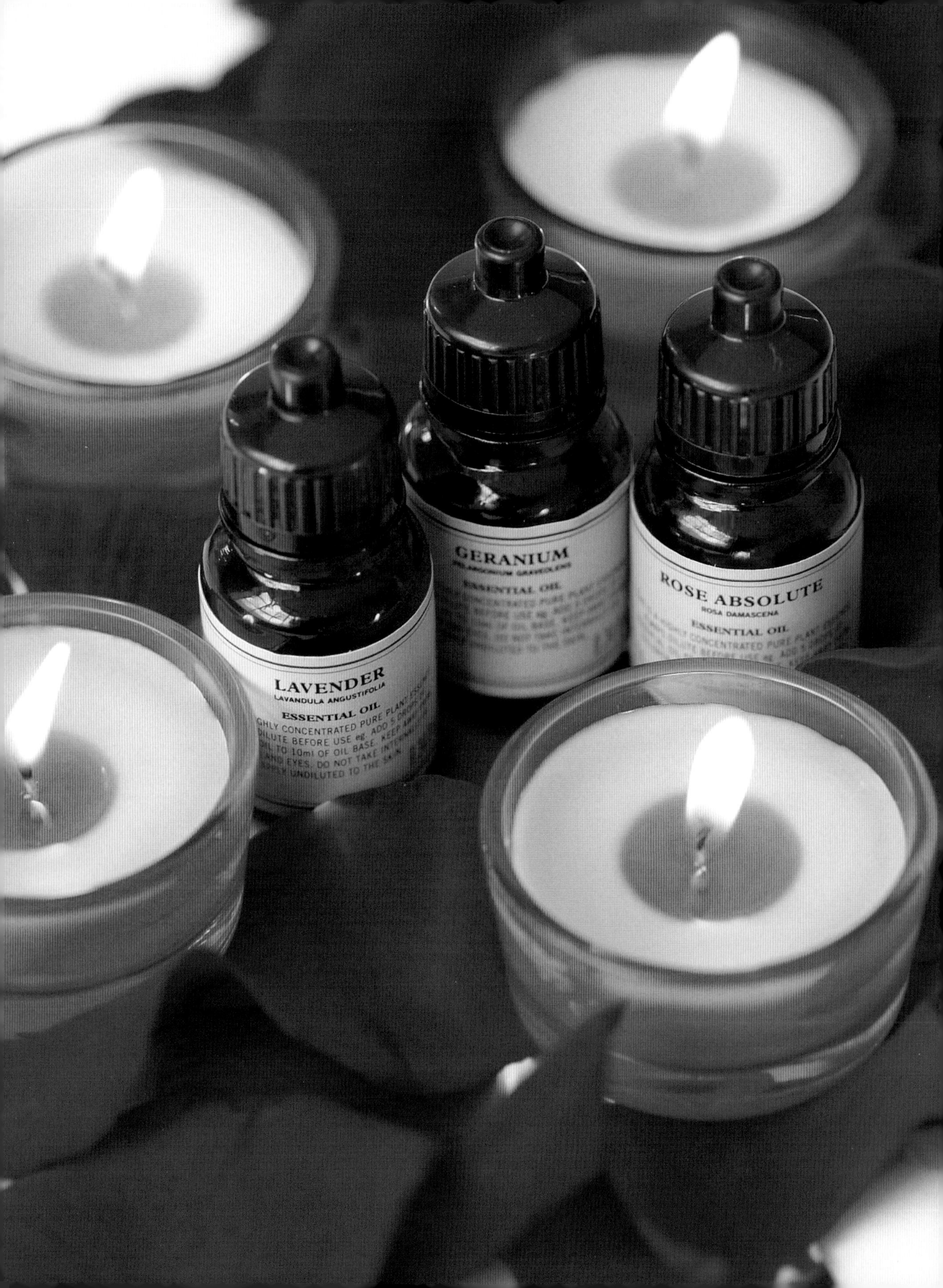
GERANIUM
ESSENTIAL OIL
ROSE ABSOLUTE
ROSA DAMASCENA
ESSENTIAL OIL
LAVENDER
LAVANDULA ANGUSTIFOLIA
ESSENTIAL OIL

to my bed for those nights when I'm just too hyper to relax. Sprayed onto the pillow, the light perfume is wonderfully soporific.

- *Rose*, one of the finest essential oils, has a powerful effect on the circulatory, digestive and nervous systems, and is especially good on mature skins.
- *Geranium* can stimulate the senses and reduce anxiety and fatigue. Some therapists believe it can also be used to help relieve menopausal problems.
- *Jasmine* is sometimes described as the 'woman's best friend'. Its aroma is often used to help menstrual cramps and the physical discomforts of the menopause. It's also supposed to induce confidence, is an anti-depressant and, in some cultures, is used as an aphrodisiac.
- *Neroli* comes from the flowers of the bitter orange and can reduce muscle spasms and help stimulate the growth of healthy new skin, so it's especially good for mature skin that's been damaged as the result of an accident or illness.

Shiatsu

This is a form of massage developed in Japan in which pressure is applied to points on the body similar to those used in acupuncture. It works on the principle that energy (or *chi*) flows through the body and when that flow is blocked the whole body is out of balance. To restore the flow the masseur applies pressure to the relevant points on the body.

Self-massage

You're never going to be able to give yourself a complete body massage, but there are parts of the body within easy reach that will benefit from regular attention. It helps your circulation, releases tension and eases pain. Before you start, make sure you apply massage oil or cream to your hands in generous amounts to help them slide over your skin, it will be much more effective than working on dry skin. The only exception is if you massage through your clothes (as many Eastern masseurs do).

- *Neck and shoulders* Hold your right elbow in your left hand, or rest your right elbow on a solid surface to give you stability. Place your right hand on the large muscle across your shoulder and squeeze the tensions out using strong fingers. Repeat on the other side.
- *Arms* Use your thumb to squeeze into the muscle on the underside of the top of your arm, then place the palm of your hand on the top of the muscle and squeeze using your fingers, gently working up and down between the shoulder and elbow. Repeat on the other arm.

Essential oils are age-old remedies for many body ailments and can be used to lift moods, too. Aromatherapists will make special recommendations for mature skins and concerns.

- *Stomach* To help relieve bloating and constipation, place one hand on the centre of your stomach, and using the heel of your hand make small clockwise circular movements, working out from the centre to cover the whole of your abdomen. Work back into the centre and then out again, using as much pressure as you find comfortable. For a firmer massage, make a fist of your right hand, cover it with the left hand and gently press your way around the stomach in a circle putting slightly more pressure on the left side of your stomach. This will help stimulate the colon and relieve symptoms.
- *Hands* With your thumb, use firm pressure to stroke down the back of your hand between the tendons from your knuckles to your wrist. Do the same on the palm, not forgetting the area at the base of the thumb, finishing off with strong circular movements in the centre of the palm. Finally, grasp each finger in turn at the base and 'flick' the fingers up to their tips. This helps improve your circulation and eases any aching joints. Repeat on the other hand.
- *Feet* As with the hands, use your thumb to work up through the tendons towards the fleshy bit just below the arch of the foot. Turn your foot over and use a strong thumb to make circular movements all over the sole of your foot. Grab hold of your toes and flex them backwards and forwards. Then make a fist of your hand and, using the knuckles, knead into the arch of your foot from heel to sole. Finally, grab each toe and gently pull as you 'flick' each one from base to nail. Repeat on the other foot

If you have difficulty reaching your feet, here's a simple alternative: get hold of an old tennis ball – or any ball of that size that's fairly firm – put it under your feet, and roll backwards and forwards for about a minute. Or, get a foot massager from any chemist or health store. They tend to be wooden frames set with rubber rollers that have small, round nobbles on them. By rolling your feet backwards and forwards over the rollers you get a great relaxing massage with minimum effort.

Any kind of foot massage will aid your circulation and help to give you healthy and happy feet (see Reflexology, page 129).

BODY MATTERS
Keeping Healthy

Sun Damage

I love the sun. For years, my idea of the perfect holiday was to pack a bikini, books and suntan lotion, head for somewhere warm and sunny and plonk myself on a beach for two weeks, then return to Britain tanned from top to toe and looking the picture of good health. Not any more. Well, not quite, anyway. I still love to lie in the sun, and like most people think I look better with a bit of colour rather than being 'pale and interesting'. But I now know enough about the long-term damage the sun can do to my skin to take sensible precautions and ensure I get a *healthy* tan rather than risk major problems.

The thing about sunlight is that it provides us with vitamin D, a vitamin that's essential for forming and maintaining strong bones and helping with the absorption of calcium. Research done in the United States showed that 50 per cent of women who suffered hip fractures were deficient in vitamin D. So post-menopausal women in particular need a daily dose of sunshine-rich vitamin D to help ward off osteoporosis. That doesn't mean you have to live in a sunny climate. Sunlight, or at least, daylight, is still available even on cloudy days, and you also get vitamin D from some foods, including oily fish. But the most effective and concentrated source comes from natural sunlight. You only need twenty to thirty minutes a day and you can get that taking a gentle walk or sitting outside having your morning cuppa.

Let's face it, we all feel so much better in the sunshine. People walk about with smiles on their faces and the continental habit of eating and drinking out of doors has brought a wonderfully relaxed atmosphere to British towns and cities. Who wouldn't prefer a sunshine-filled day to the dark, drizzly cold days of a British winter?

But, there is a darker side to sunlight, and we ignore it at our peril.

The sun produces two kinds of ultraviolet light: UVA, which sends radiation deep into the lower layers of the skin and can produce malignant melanoma, the most serious type of skin cancer; and UVB, the radiation responsible for 'burning' or tanning the skin. Too much UV radiation can also have a damaging effect on the immune system, and is definitely responsible for premature ageing of the skin. It's without doubt the main culprit when it comes to causing wrinkles.

Just take a look at the skin on your body where the sun never shines! Your bottom for instance. It may be sagging from a lack of muscle tone, but the skin there is generally quite smooth and wrinkle free because it's been protected from direct sunlight. One of my closest friends has problems with her thyroid. The medication she now takes means she daren't go out in the sun without the serious risk of breaking out in red blotches, so she covers up from head to toe, wearing hats, comfortable flowing trousers or long skirts and long-sleeved shirts. Her skin is classic English peaches and cream and, even though she's in her mid-fifties, she's hardly got a line on her face.

That regime is not for me. I still like to feel the sun on my skin, but I take sensible precautions to produce a healthy colour and reduce the risks of burning and triggering skin cancer to the minimum.

Foundation

If you wear make-up, check that it contains both UVA and UVB sunscreens, as these will be your first line of defence for your face. If you don't wear make-up, protect your skin with a moisturizer that contains a sunscreen or a sun lotion with an SPF of at least 15. It's essential during the summer and just as important during the winter. Cold winter sunshine might not contain the intense UV rays of the summer, but they are still there in the atmosphere and can do just as much damage. That's especially true if you're in a snowy location where the strength of the rays is intensified by reflection.

Sunbathing

As a teenager I can remember that I and all my friends in Plymouth slathered our skins with a combination of olive oil and vinegar – the oil to tan us, the vinegar to colour our skins. We must have smelt like tossed salads and roasted nicely like sausages on a grill. Nowadays there's no excuse to burn. Use a lotion that's at least SPF 15. It will protect your skin from the burning effects of the sun, and ensure you get a slow, even tan that will last much longer than the 'burn and peel' cycle you may have survived in your youth.

Apply cream at least fifteen to twenty minutes before going out in the sun to give it time to establish on your skin, and replenish it at least every two hours – more often if you are gardening, swimming, or involved in some sporting or energetic activity.

Avoid being in sunlight between 11 a.m. and 3 p.m., when the sun's rays are directly overhead and at their strongest. If you can't avoid that, then ensure you cover up with light, loose clothing, or slather on cream of a higher SPF factor. Don't forget to keep your hands well covered in cream. Excessive sun exposure is the main cause of brown age spots (see page 108).

If you're spending a day out in the sun with grandchildren or other younger members of the family, make sure they are adequately protected. I know it's great to see children running about on the beach with a good healthy brown colour, but the greatest amount of damage is done to young skin and you often don't see the results until later in life. My legs are now permanently mottled with brown freckles and white blotches where the pigmentation has disappeared, the legacy of severely burning my shins on holiday in Greece in my twenties. Keep babies out of the sun altogether – their skins are far too delicate to survive the attack of radiation – and make sure that children wear hats and a high-factor sun cream at all times. Pop them into a cotton T-shirt if the sun gets really strong, though that's good advice whatever your age.

Wear a Hat

It will give the back of your neck protection and keep the strongest rays of the sun off your face. Sun hats can also look incredibly glamorous, and hide a multitude of 'summer hair' sins.

Wear Sunglasses

They'll protect your eyes from sun damage and stop you from screwing up your face against the glare of the sun – another great wrinkle promoter.

After Sun

Always drench your skin in after-sun cream at the end of a day's sunbathing or any outdoor activity. It will be dry, parched and desperate for a drink. The ingredients will also help soothe and cool skin that's been exposed to the burning effect of the UV light.

Sunburn

If your skin is slightly burned, get into a very cool bath or take a shower as cold as you can bear it to bring down the surface temperature, then apply calamine lotion (a good old-fashioned cure) or an aloe vera after-sun gel. If you are badly burned, you must see a doctor.

Men and Sunlight

What is it about men and suntan lotion? My father was classic. He simply refused to wear any form of sun protection. He claimed he went through the war in the Pacific, often stripped to the waist, without any creams, and if it was good enough for him then, it was good enough for him now! Well, he was lucky. He had no major skin problems, and finished each summer with skin the colour and texture of an old walnut. But I cringe every time I see men lying in the sun turning a vivid and painful-looking lobster red just because they've decided that it's 'sissy' to wear sun protection. *It isn't!*

In Australia, where skin cancer affects one in four of the population, I'm told the lifeguards on the Aussie beaches have the right to insist you put on sun cream if they think you're not properly protected. No problems with infringing an individual's human rights there. They stand over you until you cover up. I suggest you do the same to your partner if he's reluctant to be sensible. Use whatever feminine trick it takes – but do it.

Skin Cancer

There's no getting away from it, excessive exposure to UV rays is a primary cause of skin cancer. It can produce new melanoma on the skin, or trigger a response in an existing mole (see pages 32–3). If you have a mole, or suddenly acquire a brown melanoma that has irregular edges, is itchy, weeping, or takes on the appearance of a wound that will not heal, you must consult your doctor immediately. Malignant melanoma can be treated if caught early, but if left, the cells will invade the rest of the body and spread to other organs.

Sunlight is a wonderful thing. All human life thrives on it. But it must be treated with respect. So if you're *really* desperate to get a deep, bronze tan, get it out of a bottle. You'll beat the wrinkles and the risk of skin cancer, and no one need know but you!

Joints

If we think of our bodies as a huge machine, then our joints are the equivalent of all the sockets and moveable bits that keep that machine turning. Lack of use, excess pressure or failing to oil the joints regularly will cause the machine to grind to a halt as everything gradually seizes up. That's exactly what happens to our bodies. Starve the joints of lubricants, leave them lying idle, or increase the pressure through excess weight, and suddenly you loose flexibility and movement and start to experience pain. The 'use it or lose it' principle applies to muscles as well as joints, but taking regular exercise and eating a good well-balanced diet will help keep the joints mobile and pain free. And it's pain that will make you a prisoner. It will limit your freedom and prevent you from doing all the things you want, from playing football with the grandchildren to enjoying days out with your friends and family and a whole host of activities in between.

Controlling your weight is also important. Our joints can only carry so much. When I was filming at an obesity clinic in an American university some years ago, I met two women who had gained so much weight their legs could no longer support their bodies and they had to move around on electronic buggies. They weren't disabled in the medical sense of the word, just too fat to walk. They were extreme cases, but a reminder that excess weight can not only pose real health problems, but also impose major limitations on your mobility and the freedom to get the most out of life.

For years now, I've started every day with a ten-minute routine of stretching and bending, using exercises based on simple yoga movements, to iron out the kinks in my body from a night's sleep, and most importantly to keep my joints mobile, supple and strong. It means I can get on with my life without being slowed down by stiffness or held up by pain. You'll find a few simple exercises in Chapter Thirteen which should be helpful.

There's a saying in the dance world that if you miss ballet class for one day you notice the effect, if you miss two days, your colleagues notice, and if you miss three days, the audience notices. That's because dancers' bodies are so well honed that the minute they stop using them, the joints and muscles begin to seize up. I know myself that if for any reason I skip a couple of mornings and don't go through my routine, or miss out a couple of exercises, when I come back to it, my body feels a little more stiff, and takes a few days to loosen up again. So just think what happens when you don't work your joints for several years! But it doesn't have to be too late. Spending a few minutes

every day loosening up joints will help promote the body's natural lubricants, and you can help it by taking a daily fish oil supplement or glucosamine (see pages 153–4).

I remember a few years ago a woman in her sixties, who joined a yoga class I attended, could barely bend to touch her knees when she started. A year later, with steady and careful progress, she was touching the floor with straight knees and a strong, supple back. We all cheered the first time she did it, and the look on her face was priceless. So don't expect an overnight transformation, but keep at it, and your body will be freed-up and raring to go.

Circulation

Poor circulation can lead to all sorts of problems with your body: from angina, heart attacks and strokes at one end of the spectrum, to cold feet, poor skin condition, cellulite, cramps and dep vein thrombosis (DVT) at the other.

Menopausal women often suffer a tingling sensation in their hands and feet as the result of poor circulation, and diabetics have more problems than most, suffering from cold extremities and the risk of skin ulcers.

Massage and skin brushing can help, as discussed on pages 83–4 and 88–92, while a diet rich in antioxidants like vitamins A, C and E, and the minerals selenium (see Chapter Eleven), zinc and manganese will help keep the arteries clear. Ginger and garlic in your food are wonderful natural stimulants for the circulation. For an instant pick-me-up on cold days grate a little root ginger into a cup of hot water and add a dash of honey. It's also a great tummy settler if you feel bloated.

But there's really no better way of improving your

circulation than taking some form of regular exercise (see Chapter Thirteen). It will keep your joints mobile and your body healthy because you increase the oxygen supply to your blood and encourage your heart and muscles to pump it around your body. Find the level of exercise that suits your lifestyle and general health and never take on any form of extra exertion without checking with your doctor first. Once you've got the all-clear, embark on something you can really enjoy and are able to do regularly. It may be dancing, going to the gym, swimming or just going for a brisk thirty-minute walk three times a week. Whatever you choose, make sure it's something you're going to enjoy, or it will be too easy to find excuses to give up. If you're house-bound, or have limited mobility, check out some of the exercises in Chapter Thirteen. Even a small amount of movement is better than none at all, and it's amazing what your body can get up to just sitting in a chair!

Exercising will help to de-stress you (especially if you choose something like Pilates, yoga or t'ai chi) and ease all manner of aches and pains as your muscles become stronger and your joints more mobile. On those days when you feel drained of all energy get out a skipping rope and give yourself a steady ten-minute workout, or find a music station or favourite recording that supplies music with a solid dance beat. Bop around for ten or fifteen minutes and your energy levels will soar. My instant pick-me-up is the sound track from the film *The Full Monty*. With or without the strip at the end, it gets me moovin' and groovin' and feeling great.

Cellulite

Although most women associate cellulite with their thighs and buttocks (see pages 112–5), it can creep into other parts of the body, especially around the waist and tummy. The problem is the same – pockets of fat sitting stubbornly in sluggish body cells – so the solution is the same – break it up and move it out. Gentle body brushing, exercise, diet and drinking lots of water should still form your main attack strategy, but if more drastic action is needed try one of the salon treatments on page 115.

Surgical Solutions

Surgical solutions for problem areas like tummies, hips and breasts are included in Chapter Nine.

Listen to your body. It will tell you when it needs help because it's dry, over-tired, wearing out or breaking down. Don't ignore the warning signs it sends out. They won't go away, and could get worse. So when the alarm bells start ringing, even if they're only very quiet, consult your doctor or get help from a specialist therapist. Once you know how your body feels when it's fit and well, you'll feel so good about yourself you'll want to keep it that way for as long as possible.

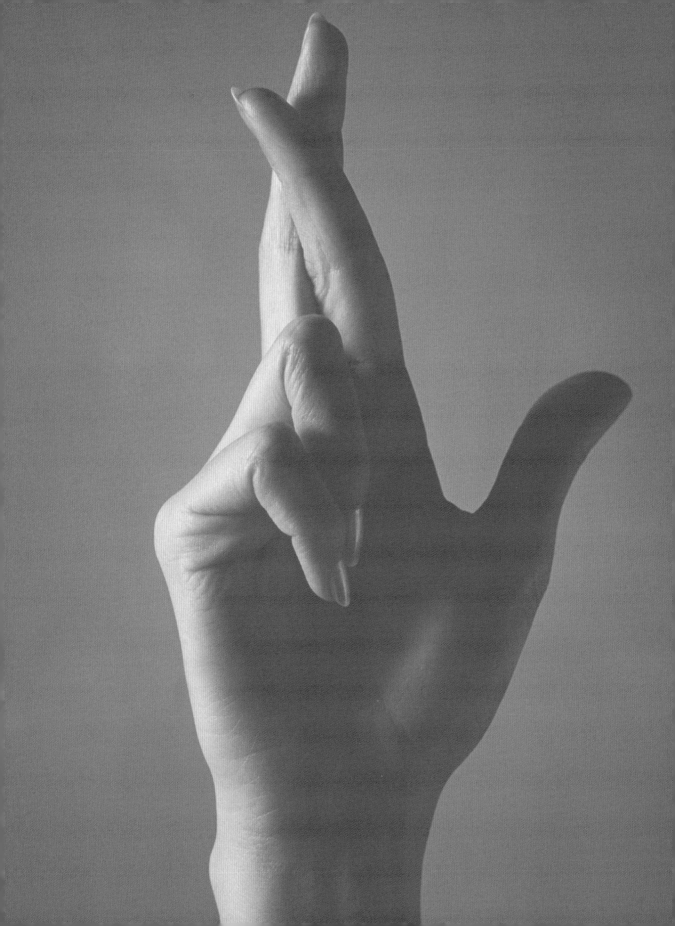

6
HANDS AND NAILS

There's no bigger giveaway to a woman's age than the appearance of her hands. You can have all the anti-ageing treatments in the world on your face, and keep a trim youthful body shape with good diet and exercise, but if you haven't taken care of your hands, they'll show the passage of time more blatantly than any other part of your body. Just think about Jane Fonda, or Nancy Reagan, or indeed any woman you know with a surgically enhanced face or a body that testifies to years of strict health regimes. They probably look great for their age, but once they put their hands anywhere near their faces, or start talking with their hands, chances are you'll add about ten years to the date you *thought* was on their birth certificate.

I've always had very soft nails that break or chip just opening a drawer, and my veins stand out like an aerial map of the Ganges delta, so I'm never going to be able to fool anyone about how old I am. Besides, I went to school with too many girls who have long memories and big mouths to lie about my age, so I just do my best to keep my hands in good condition and hope they don't look any worse than they have to.

HANDS AND NAILS
Keeping Young and Beautiful

Unlike the rest of our body, where we can cover imperfections with make-up or clothes, our hands are constantly on show. But achieving soft, well-groomed hands and nails doesn't have to be either time consuming or expensive, and the result can be such a confidence booster. I always think there's something wonderfully defiant about seeing a flash of colour on an older woman's hand. I've met women in their eighties and nineties with wonderfully expressive hands wearing drop-dead gorgeous colours on their nails. It's as if they're saying, 'OK, I may no longer be in the first flush of youth, but I still enjoy being a truly feminine woman!'

Protection

This is essential, and means wearing gloves whenever you do any housework, gardening, or manual task that brings your hands into contact with water or abrasive substances. When you're gardening, a layer of barrier or hand cream will give you extra protection against the drying and scouring effects of the soil. You should also always wear warm gloves in the winter to help your circulation and protect your hands from the drying effects of cold weather.

Hand cream will keep the skin moisturized, supple and protected. Keep a tube next to every sink and washbasin in the house, and get into the habit of *always* applying a little cream whenever you've washed your hands. It doesn't have to be a huge dollop, and it certainly does not have to be expensive. Always apply hand cream last thing at night, when it has several hours to soak in without work or water to disturb it.

Sun damage is a primary cause of skin ageing anywhere on the body. We tend to forget just how much exposure our hands get to ultraviolet light throughout the year, so it's really important to cover them with sun cream whenever you go out – even if all you're doing is walking the dog or

Hands that are in desperate need of moisture will benefit from an overnight dose of vaseline. Slather it on last thing at night, and then wear a pair of cotton gloves to encourage warmth and help absorption, not to mention keeping the petroleum jelly off the bedclothes! (The Body Shop sells them.) By morning your hands will be unbelievably soft.

going shopping – especially during the summer. Overexposure to UV light leads to age or liver spots. They're not freckles, they're a direct result of sun damage. Wearing an SPF 15 sun cream is your best protection against further damage, and most hand creams now contain both sun screens and hydroquinone, which will help fade existing spots. But once you have them, the only sure way of eliminating them is by zapping them with a laser, which is something that a good cosmetic surgeon should be able to do.

Cosmetic Surgery

Surgery or anti-ageing treatments can be applied to most parts of the face and body, but the hands don't respond to 'lifts and tucks' in the same way as the face or tummy.

If, like me, you have soft nails that split or snap easily, always carry an emery board with you. If you can get to the damage quickly and file the nail into a smooth outline, it will avoid the temptation to pull the nail off and ruin the shape.

Apart from using a laser to remove brown age spots, there are really only two effective treatments for ageing hands. The first is a fat injection to plump-up the skin and smooth out the effect of the prominent veins. The fat is taken from your own body, usually around the hips or thighs, so there is no problem with cross infection or rejection. It can be done under local anaesthetic in less than an hour, although top cosmetic surgeon Dai Davies is not convinced it gives anything more than a short-term benefit.

The other treatment is a skin peel. Using the same laser technology that removes skin from the face in treatments to reduce wrinkles, it's possible to laser off the top layer of skin and encourage new, plumper skin to grow to the surface (see Face Peel, page 138). However, here's a word of caution from Dai Davies, 'Overall, these treatments are disappointing and not widely practised by reputable surgeons in the UK.'

Hand Scrubs

Use one to exfoliate dead and dry skin. This is just as important in maintaining soft hands as the exfoliation regime that keeps the rest of your skin in good shape. When you use an exfoliant in the bath or shower, remember to give your hands the treatment as well, or use a specific hand scrub, like the one produced by the French company L'Occitane. The combination of wheatgerm and clay helps to clean and draw out impurities, leaving the skin wonderfully soft, as well as slightly fading age spots. On really rough hands the Crabtree and Evelyn Gardener's Hand Scrub with Pumice does a great job of restoration. Or use our old favourite, salt.

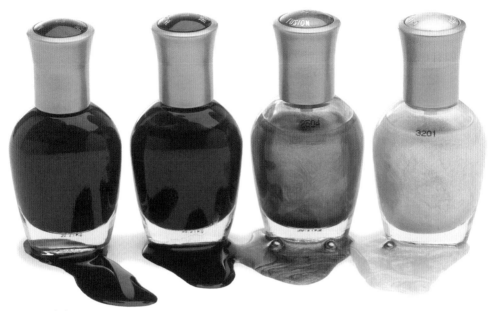

Massage

Massage encourages good circulation and helps keep your hands supple as well as healthy (see page 92). Many hospitals, hospices and care homes now include hand massage and nail care as part of their regular regimes, having recognized the feel-good factor they produce.

Manicures

Treating yourself to a regular manicure is a wonderful way of spending a relaxing half hour or so, and the transformation to your hands can be pretty dramatic. I always think that soft hands and well-manicured nails make a woman look well groomed and feminine and, because our hands are constantly on show, that can be a great confidence booster. Once you start worrying about chipped nails and rough hands it can really cramp your style in public.

A little almond oil or a specific cuticle cream or oil massaged into the nail bed every evening will help keep the cuticles soft and feed the nail bed, encouraging stronger nails.

I think one of the great exports from America over the past few years has been the introduction of walk-in nail parlours on the high street. I remember strolling through Manhattan a few years ago and thinking that every block seemed to have its own team of manicurists. It took a while for the trend to catch on here, but now that it has, there's really no excuse for not getting a professional manicure on a fairly regular basis, rather than thinking of it as an occasional, special outing.

A good manicurist should not only do a great job on your nails, she should also exfoliate and nourish your hands and make sure you have no allergic reactions to any of the things she's about to use on your skin. Acetone can be really drying on soft or mature nails, and many women are allergic to formaldehyde, so check on the ingredients of the polish before you choose a nail colour.

Keep your hands out of water for two hours after a manicure because water makes the varnish peel. Avoid hot water if you want the manicure to last longer. Wear gloves as a protection when doing the dishes or the housework.

Home Manicure

Keeping your nails in shape at home is one of the things you can do in the 'be nice to yourself' category. It's soothing and therapeutic, and because you can't really rush any part of the process it's a great way of de-stressing.

- *Start by removing any old polish* with an oil-based remover.
- *Rinse the nails* to clean off any residue of remover, *then soak your fingers* in warm water to which you've added a little baby oil or wheatgerm oil. This will soften up the cuticles and any hard patches of skin or calluses.
- *Remove hard skin, gently*, using a pumice stone, and *exfoliate the hands* either with a specific cream, or by using a combination of olive oil and salt. Rinse and dry.
- *Apply a hand cream*, really working it into the skin, and giving yourself a hand massage at the same time (see page 92).
- Using an emery board (never a metal file – they are much too harsh) *shape the nails*. Don't saw at them, because this will make the edges rough and liable to flake. File in one direction, from the edge to the centre.
- *Apply a cuticle remover* and, using an orange stick tipped with cotton wool or a rubber-topped 'hoof stick', gently push the cuticle back. The cuticle protects the nail bed where the new cells are growing, so don't be too harsh on this area or you'll damage the new nail and weaken it.
- *Wash the nails* to remove any grease, and dry them gently.
- If your nails are ridged, don't be tempted to file the ridges level, which will only weaken the nails further. *Apply a ridge filler* to even out the surfaces of your nails.
- Even if you don't intend to wear a coloured nail varnish, *apply a clear base coat* on your nails which works in much the

Nails that are soft and tend to flake need an extra boost of calcium. You should be consuming between 700–1000 mg a day. If you're not getting enough naturally from calcium-rich foods like dairy products and sardines, take a calcium citrate supplement, and make sure you also get plenty of vitamin D from sunlight to help your bones and nails achieve maximum absorption. Keep the nails short, and coat them with a nail strengthener.

same way as a conditioner does on your hair. It nourishes and protects the nails and helps prevent them from becoming brittle. It also helps stop the colour being absorbed by and staining your nails. I rarely use a colour on my nails to avoid drawing attention to them, but it's at this stage that I apply a nail strengthener. Because my nails break so easily I tend to keep them short, and then give them a bit of extra protection with something like Sally Hansen's Diamond Strength or the Barielle Nail Strengthening Remedy.

- *If you're using a colour, apply two coats,* allowing the first coat to dry for ten minutes before applying the second. Don't overload the brush. Paint the first strip of colour down the centre of the nail, then work either side.
- *Paint over the tips of your nails* – that will help to prevent chipping. Then finish off with a colourless top coat for extra protection. I find the new Autograph range of varnishes from Marks and Spencer are really long-lasting and resistant to chipping, especially if you finish off with a clear top coat.
- *Keep the top coat handy.* If and when the varnish chips and you need a quick touch up of colour, the top coat will help bind the new varnish to the nail and even out the join.

False Nails

'Falsies' are an instant route to glamour, but beware of the glue. Wear them too often, or be over-energetic in removing the nails, and you could do long-term damage to your own mature nails which may already be thin and vulnerable with ageing.

Nail extensions are best done by an expert, but again be wary of having the acrylic extensions glued to your nails too often. The natural nail needs to breathe to stay healthy. Unless you have quite exceptional hands, don't be tempted to wear your false nails too long or they could end up looking like talons!

Never shake your nail-varnish bottle. It allows small pockets of air to be trapped in the varnish, which will make it thicken prematurely. Rub the bottle between your hands; this keeps the air out, and the warmth of your hands will thin the lacquer slightly, making it easier to apply.

Yellowing nails can result from wearing dark-coloured nail lacquers. Soaking them in neat lemon juice for half an hour should remove the stain. But that's so boring! It's better to avoid the stain in the first place by always applying a base coat before any colour.

My manicure regime includes a treatment for the cuticles and measures to control breaking and chipping.

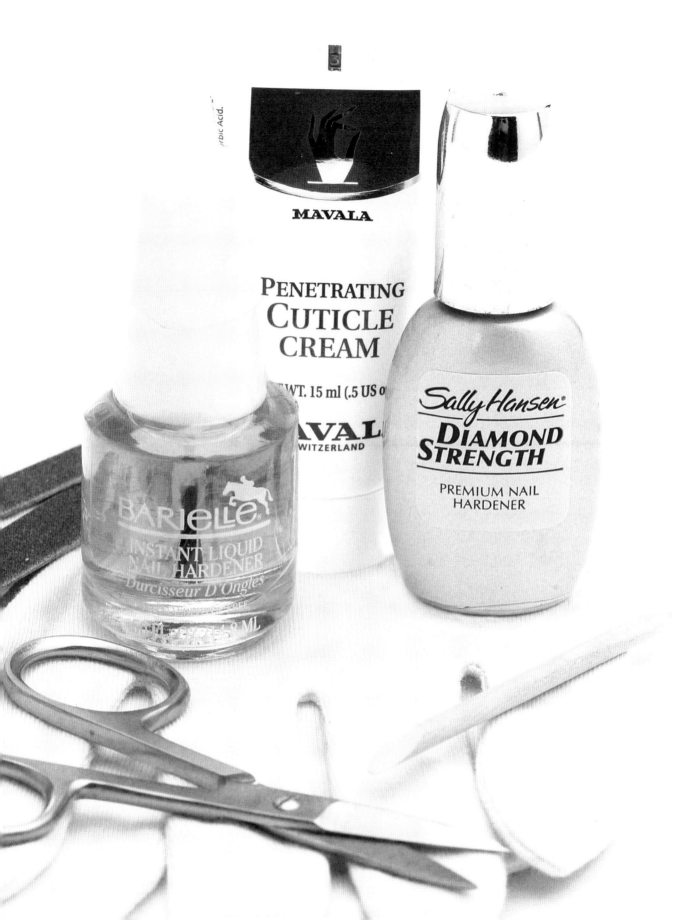

HANDS AND NAILS
Keeping Healthy

Hands are the worker bees of the body. Just think about it. They're always on the go, busy at something: tying shoelaces, dialling a telephone number, washing dishes, opening doors, knitting, writing, it's endless. In a single day they can be called upon to pick up heavy weights or apply the gentlest of touches, and perform a thousand and one tasks and movements from the smallest, seemingly inconsequential thing, like turning the page of a book or threading a needle, to the real heavyweight jobs of digging the garden or unscrewing a tight-lidded jar. Every single action involves using most of the twenty-seven bones in the hands, so over a lifetime the joints make countless millions of movements. Is it any wonder then that eventually they start to wear out and develop the pain or discomfort associated with osteoarthritis?

The irony is that if we stop using, or exercising, our hands, the joints will start to fuse and seize up anyway through inactivity. It's catch-22. The advice from leading hand surgeon Rupert Eckersley is, 'Keep your hands moving and active whenever possible. We can control the pain with drugs and, in some cases, surgery. But the real answer to keeping hands healthy and mobile is – use them, and make them work.'

You'll find exercises for the hands on page 194; in the meantime, let's take a look at the most common hand-health problems.

Osteoarthritis

Arthritis comes in two main forms. One is rheumatoid arthritis, which can be hereditary, and usually occurs early in life. So if you make it to your fifties without any sign of rheumatoid arthritis you should be OK. It's not unknown, but it's uncommon for it to affect people once they're over fifty.

The main problem for the over fifties is degenerative or osteoarthritis, which is a direct result of wear and tear. I'm afraid it's an inevitable consequence of ageing. As the cartilage in the joints, especially those in the fingers and thumbs, wears away over the years, the bones start to rub against each other. That's what causes the pain. The body's response is to protect the joints and the tendons by producing extra bone cells, which show up as lumpy bits on either side of the joints, or at the base of the thumbs. Sometimes, an injury can trigger an osteoarthritic response, but in general there's no medical rhyme or reason as to why some people who are fifty plus are more likely to succumb than others. It really is just the luck of the draw.

The good news is that although, in some cases, there can be serious deformity in the joints, our amazing ability to adapt means you rarely lose the full use and mobility of your hands.

Exercise will keep the hands mobile and encourage the production of the body's natural joint lubricants. Though if, like me, you believe in helping the body by taking supplements, a daily dose of fish oil rich in omega-3 essential fatty acids and glucosamine might help. Research and medical trials have shown these can assist in maintaining, and even increasing, good lubrication in the joints in some cases (see Chapter Eleven). Rupert

Eckersley's advice is, 'Try whatever you think might help, as long as it does no harm, and you're sensible about the cost involved. If there is no improvement after three or four months, save your money.'

If pain becomes a real problem, your doctor can prescribe anti-inflammatories or painkillers. They might even suggest a cortisone injection into the joint. As I know from personal experience, that can be quite painful, even when administered with a local anaesthetic. But it works like a dream (at least it did for me) and it kept my hands pain-free and mobile for months.

In some severe cases, the only answer is a temporary, but complete, rest. A hand specialist will construct a splint to hold and protect the joint while it recovers. But once that period is over, you'll be advised to start using the hand again as much as you can. Once you can control the pain, movement really is the best all-round treatment.

> Good news for sufferers of rheumatoid arthritis (if not quite yet!). According to Rupert Eckersley, advances in the treatment of rheumatoid arthritis are becoming so sophisticated that in his opinion within twenty years the condition will be controlled to such a degree that surgery will be virtually unnecessary.

Joint Replacement

Something of a last resort this, because while the technology is improving, it's not yet as advanced as that used in say, hip or knee replacements. It will relieve pain, but do nothing to improve your range of movement.

It's impossible to replace the first joints of the finger. However, they can be fused, which will eliminate the pain, but leave you with absolutely no movement at all.

The middle joint can be replaced, and even though your range of movement may be somewhat restricted, if it's a choice between that and intolerable pain, there's really no contest.

Dupuytren's Disease or Contracture

One of the oddities of our hands, and indeed of the skin on the soles of our feet, is that on the palm, the skin doesn't move around much in the way it does elsewhere on the body. That's because the fibrous tissue is structured in such a way that it holds the skin firmly in place. With age, this tissue can start to thicken and form into either small nodules or cords that spread from the palm of the hand towards the fingers. Once the thickening reaches the fingers it starts to pull them down. It means you'll be able to make a fist, but not straighten your fingers. Try the tabletop test: if you can flatten your hand, no problem; if not, you have Dupuytren's Disease, and if it starts to bother you, there is a surgical remedy. In the past, this meant removing all the thickened tissue and covering the area with a skin graft. Nowadays it's much more subtle. A procedure known as a needle fasciotomy is done under local anaesthetic to divide and stretch the cords, allowing the fingers to return to normal. The process is much less invasive and the recovery quicker, but as the contracture is incurable, you may get a recurrence. As with so many things, surgical advances are being made all the time, so dealing with the problem of Dupuytren's is becoming fairly commonplace.

Mallet Finger

A condition in which you rupture the tendon in the fingers, making the top of the finger droop. It's easily done when you catch your fingers in something, perhaps when you're making the bed, or if you jam your finger in a door. It may seem mild, and it's easy to ignore it and assume the pain will go away in time. It won't. Early recognition means you can get the finger put in a splint, and in 90 per cent of cases it will heal. If you leave it too long, however, the finger will start to 'set' and the recovery could be less effective and take longer.

Carpal Tunnel Syndrome

There are nine tendons and one large nerve feeding into the hand and they all have to fit into that tiny space between the end of your arm and the wrist, alongside all the bones, veins and soft tissue. As you can imagine, it's pretty crowded in there, and it's not unknown for the nerve to get trapped. When that

> If you feel there's a weakness in your hand or wrist, use a bandage or surgical strap to support it, especially if you're gardening, doing heavy housework, playing sport or even carrying the shopping. And remember (especially the man in your life!), there is nothing sissy about wearing a support or strapping. Even the most macho of football and rugby players do it all the time.

happens, you start to feel pins and needles in your hand. If it's fairly mild, you may ignore it at first, but in time, if the condition worsens, you'll find you experience a significant loss of function. It'll be more difficult to do things that rely on touch, like tying shoelaces, doing up buttons, or sewing. It also becomes very dangerous because you lose sensation in the hand and increase the risk of injury through burns or cuts or trauma. In the worst-case scenario, the muscles of the hand will gradually waste away.

So don't ignore it. A simple operation can release the nerve and give you back the full use of your hands.

Trauma

Because our hands find themselves in all manner of potentially hazardous situations, the risk of damage is enormous. On the backs of the hands, where the skin is especially thin and the tendons close to the surface, a blow or cut can do serious damage. Similarly on the palm, a cut can easily slice through nerve tissue and cause numbness. So protect your hands whenever you can with protective gloves (for the washing up, gardening or manual jobs) and always be aware of their vulnerability.

Sun Damage

The sun is the main culprit for the formation of brown age spots, and there is always the risk of skin cancer (see page 32). Age spots can be reduced (see page 101), but equally they can be prevented. Why do you think our great-grannies (well, some of them, anyway) always wore lace or cotton gloves in the summer? Unless you want to start a whole new fashion craze, that's not very practical these days. But what you can do is always wear sun cream on your hands for protection in exactly the same way you put it on your face or the rest of your body. Even if you're just out shopping, your hands are exposed. So use it like a hand cream and get toasty brown rather than freckled.

Nail Lesions

Rare, but not something to be ignored. Very occasionally, you might get a problem on the side of the nail at the top of the cuticle. It will look like a small cut that weeps constantly and just won't clear up. If it persists for more than two months, consult your doctor. There's a very slight chance you have a small cancerous growth.

A clear base coat for your nails works in much the same way as a conditioner nourishes and strengthens your hair.

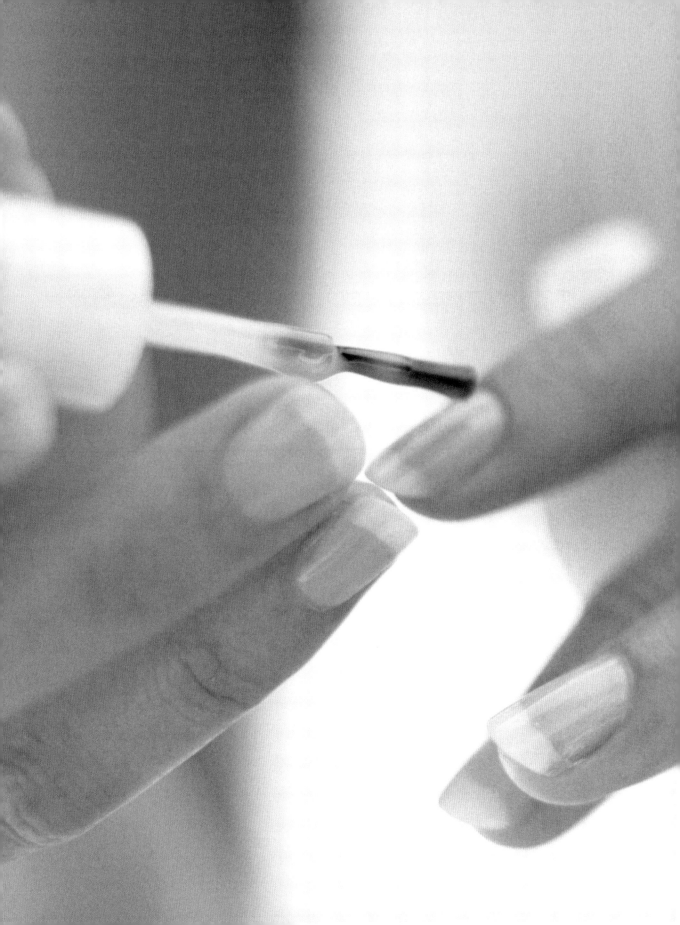

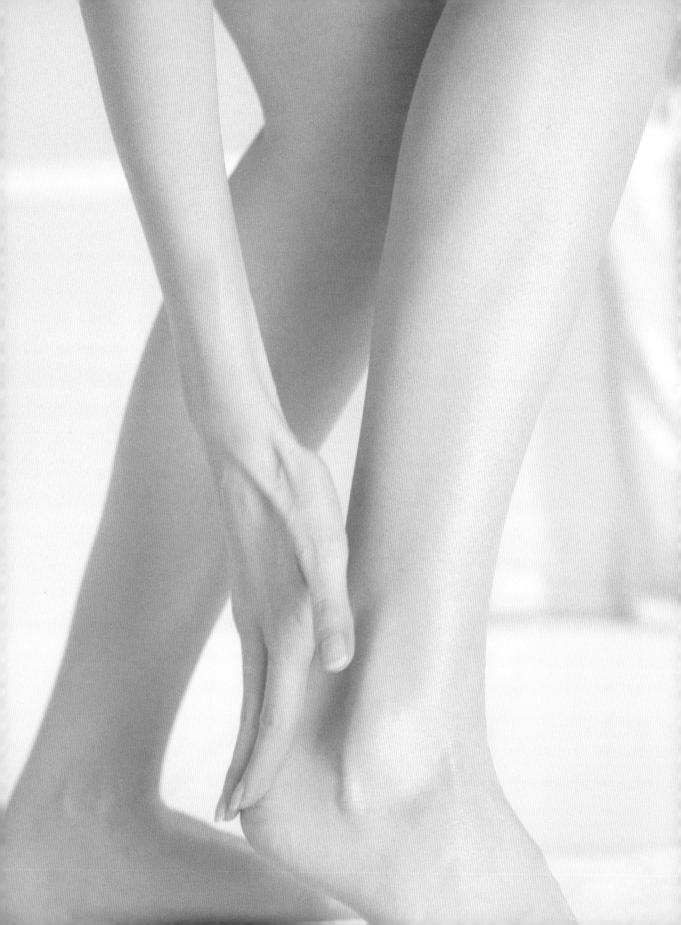

7

LEGS

Some years ago I was given a nickname by the tabloid press of 'Legs Rippon'. No prizes for guessing that it was the result of my appearance on the *Morecambe and Wise Christmas Show* in 1976 (yes, it really was that long ago!). Dancing with Eric and Ern is something I wouldn't have missed for the world because they were both such terrific guys, but it not only earned me a place in the archives of television history, it also put me firmly in the national consciousness as the newsreader with legs. Now, I don't mind the nickname, actually it's quite flattering, but as I always thought I was born with skinny legs and bony knees, I do feel a bit of a fraud.

Be that as it may, the fact that for the past twenty-five years or so I've been invited fairly regularly by assorted passing lorry drivers and various other itinerant males to, ''Ere, Ange, show us your legs,' means, I guess, that I've become more conscious of the need to keep my legs in reasonable nick than I might have been otherwise.

Certainly once I hit fifty, one thing became very clear: good legs aren't just a question of cosmetics (though regular de-fuzzing and lashings of moisturizer really do work wonders). No, the real key to having good legs is to have *healthy* legs. Legs that are free of varicose veins, thread veins and cellulite. And that goes for men just as much as it does for women, because I've noticed over the years that guys can have all sorts of nasty problems lurking in the dark under their trousers, where they reckon no one is going to see them until the summer when they venture out in shorts.

But out of sight is not out of mind, certainly not where legs are concerned. Eventually the aches and the pains associated with bad circulation and throbbing veins will take their toll on men and women alike. And cellulite is a bit like the classic unwelcome visitor: it sits there, looking a mess and won't budge until forcibly removed.

LEGS
Keeping Young and Beautiful

There's not a lot we can do with the basic shape and length of our legs. You have to be born with legs up to your armpits like Jodie Kidd or slim ankles like Betty Boothroyd. But that still leaves plenty of scope to make the best of what you *were* born with, to ensure that your legs don't just *look* lovely, they're healthy too. If you want to look great in a favourite skirt, or perhaps bare all on the beach every summer, or simply just face the next several years with comfortable, pain-free legs, start now, and before you know it, you'll be able to 'show a leg' with confidence.

So let's get to work.

Cellulite

Frankly, whoever comes up with an inexpensive, quick, simple and totally effective way of ridding our thighs, buttocks and tums of those hard, lumpy deposits for ever, will, deservedly, become a millionaire overnight.

We're all vulnerable. Regardless of age, I don't know a single woman whose body is a totally cellulite-free zone. Just look at the tabloid glee whenever a tiny spot of orange-peel skin is picked up by the paparazzi on the legs of one of the pop divas or glamour queens like Kylie Minogue.

But even if there isn't a guaranteed way of ridding your legs of cellulite for ever, don't lose heart. There's still a lot you can do to improve the situation.

Cellulite is fat that's crept into cells that aren't being worked or flushed through. It encourages other fat to join it and, because it's just sitting there doing nothing, eventually it turns into hard, lumpy deposits. The trick is to break it up and flush it out.

My top tip is to incorporate dry body brushing into your morning routine (see page 83). Use a brush with natural bristles. Origins make a fabulous one out of coconut fibre, though I've also used an old, natural-bristle hairbrush. On dry skin, before you bathe or shower, start at the ankles and make long sweeps, up the legs (always towards the heart),

All is not lost if you find yourself with orange-peel skin. Get bodybrushing and exercising, and keep an eye on those toxins.

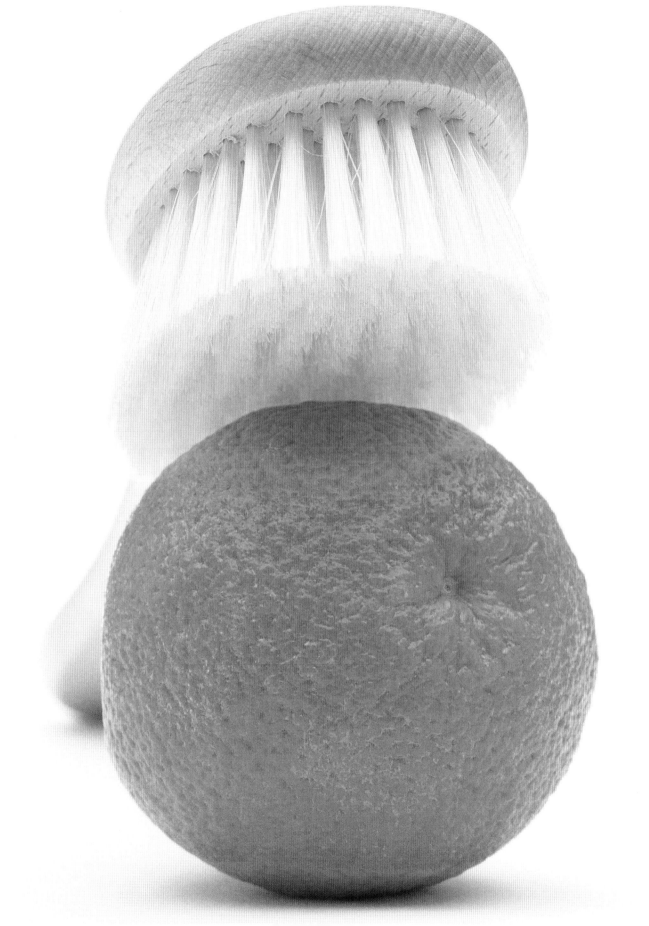

and pay particular attention to the inner and outer thighs, the insides of the knees and the buttocks. This stirs up the circulation, helps break down the fat deposits, and encourages lymphatic drainage. The flow of lymph is the body's natural waste-disposal system, as it races through the cells it drives out toxins and picks up globules of unwanted fat. By starting at the ankles, you also help to eliminate waste around the feet and discourage puffy ankles.

Make just a few strokes to start with, and use only a light pressure. As your body becomes more used to the sensation you can increase both the frequency of the strokes and the pressure. If you have varicose veins or ulcers, avoid them totally. Dry brush only on skin that is blemish- and vein-free.

Do this regularly and you'll notice a three-way bonus: in addition to improved lymph drainage, your circulation will improve and you'll be sloughing off old dead skin cells, so your skin will look brighter and feel smoother. It won't happen overnight, but in time you'll notice a real difference to the texture of your skin, and a reduction in the fatty deposits.

Drink Pure Water

Just as you use lots of water to flush rubbish down the sink, so you need at least 1.5 litres of still water a day to flush waste and toxins out of the body. The water in tea, coffee and fruit juices doesn't count, unless you're drinking herb tea or green tea, which is full of antioxidants. It has to be plain water, preferably without gas, which the human body was never designed to accommodate.

Exercise

Exercise is important. It can be anything that makes the legs really work, like cycling, swimming or walking. It doesn't have to be exhausting. A brisk walk, rather than a gentle stroll, when you're out with the dog or going to the post office will do. But if you can manage thirty minutes three times a week, that should be your goal. If you want a role model, look no further than Tina Turner. She's in her sixties and still has fabulous legs. That's because for years she danced non-stop during her stage shows. Cellulite didn't stand a chance.

Cellulite Creams and Treatments

There are numerous anti-cellulite creams and gels on the market, all claiming to 'help reduce the appearance of orange-peel skin'. Chemists will tell you they are nothing more than a promise in a pot and that ridding your body of cellulite takes a lot more than just rubbing in a cream. What I've found is that they do help improve the condition of the skin, while the mere act of massaging the cellulite tones the body and does help in breaking down the fatty deposits, but don't really expect more than that.

Salon Treatments

Beauty salons offer a whole range of pummelling, vibrating, seaweed wrapping and muscle-stimulation treatments to attack the cellulite.

They do eventually improve the appearance of the skin, but all of them require a significant investment of time and money.

General Maintenance

Moisturize

I can't emphasize enough how important it is to moisturize your legs with a body cream every morning. The skin over your shins is especially thin and prone to go dry, wrinkled and flaky if ignored. So slather on the cream daily, taking it down over your ankles and onto your heels to minimize the effects of dry hard skin. Massage well into your calves and between any protruding veins to help stimulate circulation.

De-fuzzing

Shaving

The quickest, and for many women, the easiest way of keeping legs hair free is to shave, though the effect doesn't last as long as some other methods.

A word of advice: don't be tempted to use your husband's or partner's razor. It may not always be as sharp as you want, men do tend to get a bit grumpy if we clog up the blades with our longer hairs and, frankly, it's downright unhygienic. Buy your own. Gillette make a wonderful ladies' razor called Venus. It has a double blade on a floating head (all the better for negotiating feminine curves) and a handle that's ergonomically designed to fit comfortably into your hand.

Resist the temptation to 'dry' shave, without any form of soap. The blades will cut into the top layer of skin cells and make the skin decidedly sore with razor burn. I know, I've done it! Use a shaving foam or soap to soften up the skin, and more importantly soften up the hairs. Dry hair is as tough as a piece of wire, but once it's exposed to heat and

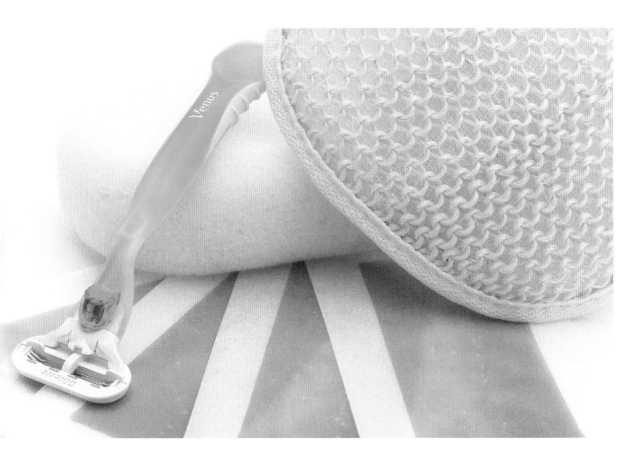

water, it becomes easier to shave. That's why an old-fashioned barber always wraps a man's face in a hot towel before he begins shaving him.

Use long, gentle strokes without too much pressure on the blade. Overdo it and you'll cut yourself. Don't forget the knees, where you can get quite a spiky growth making them look like mini hedgehogs, and then work your way up to the bikini line.

For me, there is nothing more ugly and unfeminine than seeing a woman, of any age, in a bathing costume with a fuzz of hair sprouting from her crotch (unless it's underneath her arms, which is just as bad!). Again, use lots of soap or foam, and gently pull the skin at the crotch a little taut before you begin to shave to reduce the risk of nicking loose skin.

Always finish off with a light application of moisturizing lotion to counter any possibility of razor burn.

Cream Depilatories

These work by promoting a chemical reaction on the hair, which dissolves it just below the surface so you can then either wash off the cream and unwanted hair, or remove it with a spatula. It's probably the best way to de-fuzz heavily veined legs.

Waxing

Usually done in a salon, this is one of the most effective and long-lasting ways of removing hair from the legs and bikini line. Hot wax is spread over the hairs, allowed to cool, and then torn off using a muslin cloth. It can be painful because the hairs are literally torn out of their follicles. But you're left with wonderfully smooth skin, and hair-free legs for several weeks. Cost will vary according to the salon you use, but an average price would be about £9.00 for a bikini wax, £17.00 for a half leg (up to the knee) and £28.00 for a full leg and bikini wax. Nowadays several manufacturers like Veet have produced really easy to use home-waxing kits. In the past, they tended to be messy and time consuming, but now you can roll on the wax from a dispenser with a roller ball similar to the one you have on a deodorant. They should not to be used on broken skin or areas badly affected by prominent veins.

Wax Strips

This is the easiest way to wax off unwanted hair at home. The strips are coated with a gluey substance and you simply press them onto the skin, and then rip them off in the opposite direction to the hair growth. Satisfyingly quick and clean, the strips produced by Jolen and Boots are really effective. Again, don't attempt to use them on damaged skin.

Fake It

Legs always seem to take for ever to brown in the summer. So if you want to go without tights or stockings, but can't stand the sight of two pasty white sticks peeking out from skirts and shorts, apply a fake tan and give yourself a glorious bronzed look in no time at all. It's also a lot healthier to fake it rather than to sit in the sun for hours.

To get the best effect, exfoliate the legs first, and then moisturize. This will give you a really good base to work on and help the fake colour spread evenly without streaking.

LEGS
Keeping Healthy

Varicose Veins: A Few Preventative Measures

Veins start to become problematical and lumpy when the valves, which are supposed to keep the blood flowing upwards towards the heart, grow weak, malfunction and allow the blood to drop back down the legs forming 'puddles' in the calf or behind the knee.

All sorts of things can be responsible for this happening, from being overweight to having poor circulation. Hormonal changes during the menopause can affect your legs, as can the after-effects of pregnancy. It may be some time since you had your children, but the long-term effects of carrying that extra weight for nine months can take years to develop fully. So if you've reached fifty-plus and are still free of problematical veins, you want to keep it that way. But, if you've recently started to get achy legs and have noticed a few telltale blue or red lines, it's not too late, because there are things you can do to ensure the situation doesn't get out of control.

Some form of exercise that really works the leg muscles, especially those in the calf, is essential (see Chapter Thirteen). Not only will this help keep the walls of the veins strong and healthy, but it will also enable the muscles in the calf to act like a pump, pushing the blood upwards and supporting any weak valves.

As proof of this, one of my regular tennis partners is eighty-two, but has the legs of a thirty-year-old man. Not a blemish on them. But then, he's been playing tennis regularly since he was a young man; the rest of us may not have that advantage. Start by taking a brisk thirty-minute walk three times a week, or try this simple exercise:

Stand on the edge of a step, something like a doorstep, or the bottom step on a flight of stairs (never the top or anywhere high in case you lose your balance and topple over). Hang on to something for support – the door-jamb or the banister. Have your toes on the step and your heels hanging over the edge with your weight pressing down. Raise your heels up and down, and feel the stretch in the calf muscles. If your legs are weak or ache, do this just ten times, but work up to thirty repetitions.

A few other simple things that will really help improve circulation and keep bulging veins and aching legs at bay are:

- *If you are sitting down for any length of time* behind a desk, in a car, train, coach or aircraft, *spend a few minutes regularly flexing your feet.* Start with them flat on the ground and raise your toes, then your heels in a rocking motion. You don't need any extra room to do this, and it's quite discreet. It's especially good advice to combat deep vein thrombosis – especially on long journeys.

- *Try to get your feet above your head for at least ten minutes a day*. Lie on the floor, perhaps with your feet on a chair. Or stretch out on the sofa with your feet propped up on the arm when watching television, or sneak a nap on the bed with your feet up on a couple of pillows.
- *Don't cross your legs when you're sitting* – try to cross your ankles instead.
- *Avoid clothes* (including underwear and tights) *that are tight across the groin* and block the flow of blood and make it harder for the valves to pump upwards.
- *Try a course of horse chestnut* (the herb aescin), which may help to strengthen the walls of the blood vessels and prevent the softening and bulging that comes with varicose veins. It might also help reduce inflammation.
- *Wear support tights or, in the winter, Lycra tights*, which are comfortable and fashionable – the gentle pressure they produce on the legs stops the blood collecting in pools.

Varicose Veins: A Medical Solution

Obviously, really bad varicose veins are a medical, not a cosmetic problem, and their treatment should be discussed with your doctor.

He or she may recommend sclerotherapy, in which a solution is injected into the vein causing it to swell, stick together and eventually shut down. The flow of blood is stopped and the vein turns into scar tissue, which disappears in a few weeks. A number of surgeons are also now using laser treatments to zap the veins and achieving much the same results as sclerotherapy.

Stripping, in which the veins are literally 'stripped' out of the legs, was for many years the preferred option for many surgeons, but for a while it was overtaken by sclerotherapy and laser solutions. However, according to a leading British vascular surgeon, it's back in favour as the most effective and successful remedy. The operation is usually done in two parts. First the complete vein between the groin and back of the knee is stripped out, then a series of small incisions is made from the knee to the ankle to remove the lower veins. You'll spend a night or two in hospital, and have your legs bandaged for about a week. Whichever method your doctor recommends, it's worth remembering that the surface veins that become varicose are not vital to us, unlike the deep veins within the legs, so losing them is really no big deal.

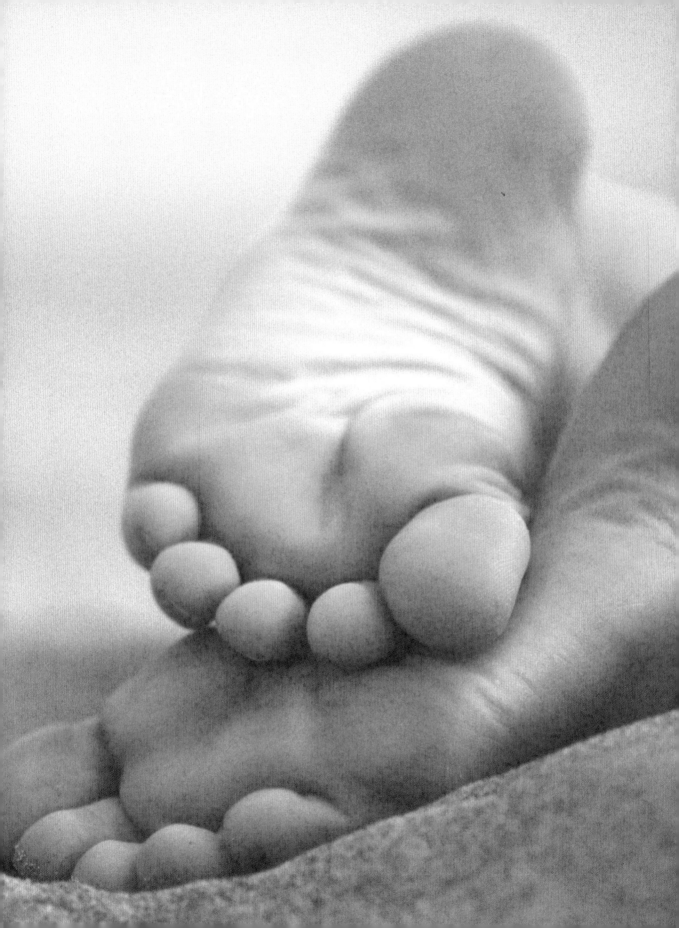

8
FEET

Feet are amazing things. They carry our whole weight around for the duration of our lives, sometimes for hours on end, over cobbled streets, hot pavements or rock-hard surfaces. They get trodden on, soaked to the skin or frozen stiff, and spend most of the year cramped up in dark, often smelly conditions. Is it any wonder they eventually start to complain? Let's face it, if feet had a union, they'd go on strike. Instead, they ache, swell up and form calluses and corns, all in the hope their owners will recognize their cry for help and occasionally give them a bit of TLC and pampering.

   We really do undervalue our feet. Perhaps their being stuck out on an extremity and wrapped up in socks and shoes, means they're 'out of sight, so out of mind'. But that's a big mistake, because badly maintained feet can have a major impact on our mobility, lower-back and knee problems, general health and pain levels. In short, all the things that can turn our journey through life into a morass of pain and discomfort rather than one marked by good health and vitality.

FEET
Keeping Young and Beautiful

Pedicures

Pretty feet are easy to achieve with regular pedicures. Being pampered by a professional technician is always a treat, but the do-it-yourself home pedicure is just as effective, if you follow a few simple rules. It's not just a case of slapping on a layer of nail polish. That may make the nails look ritzy, but won't do a lot to help the overall condition and health of your feet.

Always begin a pedicure by soaking your feet in warm soapy water. It makes them nice and clean to handle, and starts the softening-up process on the cuticles and hard skin on the heels. Right after you've had a bath is the perfect time.

Dry them well, especially between the toes, then, using a specialist foot file or pumice stone, *file away any hard skin* that's accumulated on your heels, the balls of your feet and along the sides of your big toes.

Give your feet a massage with a special foot cream. Regular hand and body creams are OK if you have nothing else, but the skin on the feet is quite different from the skin on the rest of your body and needs extra-rich emollients. Massaging will stimulate the circulation and help hydrate those areas around the heel prone to dryness.

Cuticles next. Soften them up with a special cuticle remover, and then gently push them back using an orange stick wrapped in cotton wool. Cuticles protect the nail bed from infection, so treat them with respect. If they've grown really hard don't try to cut them or pull them off; get a professional to work on them before keeping up the home maintenance.

Use nail clippers to cut your toenails straight across. Never shape them down the sides, because that can lead to ingrowing toenails. The older we get, the tougher our toenails become, especially the ones on our big toes, and clippers do a better job than scissors.

This is for when the skin on your feet is in really bad shape and you need an instant 'rescue remedy'. Slather on vaseline last thing at night, rubbing it well into the heels and soles, then put on a pair of old socks, and leave for eight hours in a warm bed to work a little miracle.

Finish off with a fine-grain nail file, but only work in one direction. 'Sawing' the file backwards and forwards will expose the fibres of the nails and make them more likely to snag and rip. To make sure they're neither too long nor too short, run your finger along the edges of your toes. If you can't feel the nails, then you've cut them too short. Always remember that the nails are there to protect your toes from being squashed or injured so they need a bit of room to do their job.

If your toenails are in poor condition, regularly massage a little almond oil into the cuticles. This will stimulate the circulation around the nail bed, and help feed the cells that are producing the new nail.

If you're going to wear polish, always apply a base coat first. Older nails are likely to be porous and will absorb the dye in lacquers, making the natural nails look yellow and unhealthy when they're bare. Two coats of colour plus a topcoat will take a good fifteen to twenty minutes to dry into a tough finish, so don't be in a rush to put your shoes on.

No matter what your age, painted toenails do look pretty, especially in the summer when your feet are bare or in sandals. Bold, dramatic colours look especially good on older feet and even if you have corns or bunions; they somehow draw attention away from the imperfections and just make your toes look pampered and feminine.

I like keeping my toenails painted all year round, even in the winter when they're tucked inside shoes or boots and no one is going to see them. You see, I reckon that painted toes are a bit like pretty underwear. They may not be on public view, but you know that underneath you're looking gorgeous.

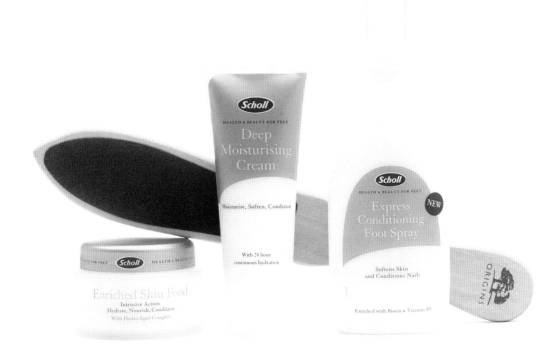

FEET
Keeping Healthy

If your feet are uncomfortable, it always shows in your face. It's hard enough trying to summon up a bright and sunny disposition if your feet are killing you, but no matter how much moisturizer you may lavish on your face to keep the wrinkles at bay, pain will etch frowns and furrows that are a dead giveaway that something is not right with the tootsies.

As any good chiropodist will tell you, most of that pain can be eliminated. According to Falguni Raja, the clinical manager at Scholl, probably the biggest name in foot care, 'Most foot problems are self-inflicted as the result of neglect. So in most cases remedies can be swift and effective, bringing almost instant relief.'

Mobility
Or lack of it, lies at the bottom of many foot problems from poor circulation to flat feet. As well as having twenty-six separate, tiny bones, the feet are a maze of muscles giving support to the whole body. If they don't get a regular workout to keep them strong and supple a number of things start going wrong.

Your circulation will be affected, leading to cold feet and skin discolouration. Because the feet are furthest away from the heart, at the end of the line as it were, they need their own pumping system to help keep the blood circulating. Without it, the toes will start to go bright pink as the blood 'pools' in the feet. The ankles will become puffy. The skin, already starved of natural collagen as part of the process of getting older, will get even more dry and flaky as it's robbed of nutrients and oxygen.

The muscles themselves will start to change shape and go flat, having lost the strength to support the arch. That's why many people find their feet spread with age – the muscles are just giving up and lying down! What happens then is that with nothing to support the arch, the foot starts to roll inwards towards the heel, throwing the whole body out of alignment. This puts pressure on the knees, the hips, the lower back and in some cases even the shoulders. The whole muscular and skeletal system is affected, bringing with it pain and discomfort. And all because the muscles in your feet have got lazy!

An immediate remedy is to have an arch or foot support fitted. A state-registered chiropodist will be able to do this having assessed your problem and recommended a suitable insole.

More long-term care and prevention means simple exercise to re-educate the muscles to work and give them strength. And don't worry – it's not that tough. Walking is the best remedy, wearing shoes that are flat, comfortable and well fitting with good, shock-absorbing soles – trainers are ideal. Aim for twenty minutes three times a week.

You don't even necessarily have to make a special time for exercising your feet. Just moving around the house, or when you're sitting down watching television, or on a car or bus journey, provide ideal opportunities for giving your feet a workout with a couple of really easy movements. You might like to try these simple exercises:

- Scrunch your toes into a 'fist' and then release them ten times.
- Write the alphabet in the air just using your feet by rotating your ankles. That will really get them working.
- Stand on tiptoe. Couldn't be easier, could it? It not only makes the muscles in your feet work, it gets the calf muscles working too, and that all helps with circulation to the feet, ankles and legs.
- You could also give your feet a treat with a regular massage. Either have it done professionally, when you see your pedicurist or chiropodist, or do it yourself (see Self-massage, pages 91–2).
- Finally, wearing exercise sandals, or walking barefoot around the house whenever possible (unless you are diabetic), gives your feet freedom and makes every muscle work.

As Falguni Raja says, 'When older people complain they don't have the mobility they used to have, quite often that just means the muscles in their feet have stopped working.'

Mobility is freedom. Freedom from pain. The freedom to go where you want, and do what you want. So give your feet a wake-up call, and get those muscles working.

The best time to buy shoes is at about 4.30 in the afternoon. Crazy but true. That's when our feet are at their biggest!

Hard Skin

The skin on the foot is quite different from the skin anywhere else on the body. It's ten times thicker for a start, and there are no sebaceous glands to keep the skin naturally lubricated, as there are elsewhere.

The combination of body weight, and the simple action of walking, concusses the skin on the heels and the soles, so in no time at all a hard ridge starts to build up to protect the bones underneath.

If the feet aren't regularly moisturized and this hard skin is left to accumulate, it will eventually cause general heel pain, and then start to crack. In the worst cases it will bleed, and lead to infection. Not a pretty sight!

Almost half the adult population suffers from hard skin on their feet, and as about 60 per cent of the population are women, the chances are that you could be one of them. So when you put this book down, pick up a foot file.

I believe everyone should have a really good foot file in their bathroom, and use it at least once a week. One of the best I've found is made by Origins. It's 27 centimetres (about 11 inches) long, so you can easily reach your feet without having to bend too much, and it's made of a solid piece of wood with a stone file set into it, which gives really firm pressure on the foot. It's a bit disconcerting to see the skin falling away like fresh chalk off a blackboard, but because the cells are dead, it doesn't hurt, and your feet will feel so much more comfortable afterwards.

When the skin is seriously cracked and inflamed, get a chiropodist to cut the dead skin away, and then keep it under control at home. Never use a blade on your own feet, it's much too dangerous.

If you're getting really hard skin on the balls of your feet, that could be because of friction or pressure from ill-fitting footwear. You might need an insole to relieve this while you're treating the hard skin.

After the filing, the pampering. Treat your feet to a massage with foot cream at least once a week. A specialist product will be rich in lanolin or paraffin wax to penetrate the thicker layers of skin, and by massaging your feet you'll do wonders for the circulation and overall condition. But don't put the cream between your toes. You don't want to give bacteria any excuse for finding a nice dark, damp breeding ground. Both Barielle and Scholl make fabulous foot creams.

Anyone not able to bend down to reach their feet could try this. Squeeze the foot cream onto the top of your left foot, then rub the bottom of your right foot over the top working it into the top and bottom of the feet at the same time. Then put the cream on the top of the right foot, and reverse the process. It's pretty much what you do when you put cream on your hands, and is good exercise for the feet too.

> To keep feet healthy and sweet, follow the chiropodist's three golden rules.
> *Smooth* using a foot file to remove all hard skin.
> *Hydrate* by massaging with foot moisturizers to keep the skin supple and aid circulation.
> *Deodorize* to reduce bacterial infection and odour.

Nail Problems

If our feet are the end of the line when it comes to circulation, then the nails are the furthermost junction off that line, and any reduction in circulation will impact directly on what happens to them. Poor circulation and a lack of nutrients will make the nails tough, especially the nail on the big toe. If they grow too long, the pressure on the nail bed as it comes into contact with footwear will cause pain and damage. Keep the nails trimmed with clippers – they're more heavy-duty than scissors.

Avoid ingrown toenails by cutting the nail straight across. If a nail does become ingrown through bad clipping or injury, bathe the foot in salt water to reduce inflammation and prevent infection; then let a chiropodist treat the problem.

Poor circulation can lead to serious disorders, with nails starting to crumble, becoming discoloured or developing fungal infections. Don't try to treat any of this yourself. Get advice and treatment from a chiropodist. If you start poking about you could worsen the condition and leave yourself open to infection.

Verrucas

These are caused by a viral infection that just loves damp places. They look like a wart, and are highly contagious. At a swimming pool or communal shower wear your own rubber flip-flops to reduce the risk of infection, and always wash your feet daily and thoroughly.

The body's own immune system will often deal with veruccas without treatment. But in feet that have poor circulation, the immune system is less effective, so a burst of liquid nitrogen from a chiropodist right onto the verruca should do the trick.

Athlete's Foot

This is an infection that thrives in the dark, damp atmosphere between the toes. Daily washing and careful drying should keep your feet clear of it. But if you develop the telltale itching and cracked skin between the toes, an anti-fungal athlete's foot powder should clear it up in a week or so. If it persists, get your doctor or chiropodist to take a look at it.

The actress Beryl Reid told me that before playing any part on stage she always had to find shoes that were exactly right for the character. Then, once her feet were comfortable, she could start building the role. Recently, the Scottish soprano Marie McLaughlin said exactly the same thng; only in her case, comfortable feet really help her to hit the high notes.

Corns

Few of us are lucky enough to go through life without ever having some sort of corn on our feet. Stilettos and winklepickers were my downfall in the sixties (yours too, I bet!). And I'm such a shoe fetishist that, when the occasion is right, I still love wearing shoes that are feminine and make my legs look good. In a toss up between vanity and short-term pain it's a no-brainer. But corns are the inevitable result of wearing anything on your feet that's too tight or restrictive. They're formed when we put pressure on the bony bits – like toes – and the body produces a plug of thick skin to relieve the pressure.

Don't ever try to cut them out yourself. You could expose the nerve endings in your toes and that's really painful. Use a corn plaster, and let the mild acid on the pad soften up the corn so you can remove it without damage to the rest of your toe. But if you are diabetic, don't ever use corn plasters; the acids on the pads could be dangerous for you. Let a chiropodist deal with the problem

Calluses

Friction or pressure help the build-up of skin that leads to calluses, and can often be a symptom of an underlying problem, like a bone deformity, style of walking or inappropriate footwear. Regular filing and moisturizing will alleviate most problems. But you may need to use a corrective insole to redistribute the pressure.

Bunions

If you've already got them I don't have to tell you that they're unsightly and painful. In simple terms they're caused by a build-up of bone, usually on the big-toe joint, though there is a similar deformity called a tailor's bunion that forms on the small-toe joint.

If they run in the family, you could be unlucky enough to have inherited the 'bunion gene', in which case you've probably had bunions since you were a teenager. For the rest of us, they're mainly caused quite simply by badly fitting shoes. Squashing our toes into narrow, tight-fitting pumps (those winklepickers again!), and forcing them downhill on high heels, plays havoc with the structure of the feet. The big toe is pushed across to the second toe, exposing the joint to pressure while bending it out of shape. Extra bone starts to build up to protect the joint, and voila, you have a bunion.

I spend a lot of my time in the company of dancers, especially ballet dancers in my role as chairman of English National Ballet. On stage, their bodies look elegant and divine, but you should see their feet! Dancing en pointe requires years of training and a pain threshold you can't imagine, as the full weight of the body is supported by toes that are crushed into the solid, confined space of a ballet shoe. Corns, bunions and bleeding toes go with the job, and once off stage, most ballerinas opt for low-heeled, wide-fitting comfortable shoes to give their feet a break. And that's the best remedy in the world.

You'll also find an arch support or a bunion pad will help to reposition your foot and relieve the pressure on the big toe. Get a chiropodist to fit it specifically to your foot, and it could make all the difference in the world.

Surgery is always an option, but most doctors only consider this when someone is in considerable pain and experiencing reduced mobility. It's rarely thought advisable for people of seventy-plus, who possibly have poor circulation or diabetes, simply because surgery could be risky. So don't leave it too late. Consult your doctor or chiropodist now. They may suggest a simple procedure in which part of the toe joint is removed and the ligaments are tightened. It can some-times lead to a floppy toe, but recovery is fairly rapid, and it's a safe option for someone who also has rheum-atoid arthritis in the joints.

A more radical approach is to take part of the bone away and insert a pin to hold it in position. You'll be in a foot cast for about six to eight weeks, and lose the flexibility in your toe.

Smelly Feet

I once came back on a flight from the South of France and sat next to a man who had the smelliest feet you can imagine. He'd taken his shoes off to be comfortable on the journey, and the stink quite put me off my plastic packed lunch. I was only grateful we were on a short hour and a half flight, and not a long haul. The interesting thing was that he obviously couldn't smell it. He was immune!

Frankly, everyone has the potential for smelly feet. There are about a 250,000 sweat glands in the feet, more than in any other part of the body, and they're all pumping out moisture throughout the day. Bacteria occur naturally in the sweat, and if left to wallow around in nice dark, damp conditions, they release an odour not unlike sewer gas.

The remedy is simple: wash your feet daily. And if you shower in the mornings, don't assume that just standing in the water is enough – it's not. Feet still need to be washed just like the rest of your body. Dry carefully between the toes and apply a foot powder. Talcum powder will help to absorb moisture, but specially formulated foot powder will soak up almost 30 per cent more moisture, so is much more effective.

Chiropodists will tell you that whenever possible you should try to avoid wearing tights or nylon pop socks, because the nylon does not absorb moisture and provides a breeding ground for the bacteria. That's really not an option for most women so, for added protection, give your feet a blast of an anti-bacterial foot spray, and make sure you rinse out your tights or socks after every wearing. If you don't, the bacteria will cling to the nylon, and be lurking there, ready to start breeding again next time you put them on.

If your feet are prone to sweating badly, carry a small spray of foot deodorizer with you for quick tops-ups during the day. It will help combat the problem, and make your feet feel much fresher. In fact, it's not a bad idea to carry one with you anyway. During a day spent shopping or sightseeing, especially in the summer, a quick spray of foot freshener is bliss for your feet, and perks you up no end.

Insoles that 'eat' odours really do work, providing

you remember to change them regularly. If you like wearing trainers, you'll know how badly they can smell after a while. Some of them will go in the washing machine without damage, but a regular zap with an anti-bacterial spray will kill off the bacteria and help keep them smelling sweeter.

Diabetes

People who are diabetic often have poor circulation. If you add this to the fact that, with age, the circulation in our feet can become sluggish, you've got a double whammy for potential problems.

If you have diabetes, it's more important than ever that you should keep your feet clean and well moisturized. Massaging foot cream all over (though not between the toes) will combat flaky skin, as well as helping to boost the circulation.

Never use corn plasters, as they contain acids which could be dangerous to you.

If your feet get cold, a common complaint with old age and poor circulation, don't be tempted to put a hot-water bottle directly on to your skin. The sensitivity in your feet will be affected and you could unwittingly burn yourself.

Finally, avoid walking barefoot. Diabetes can slow down the rate at which you heal, so you want to avoid mishaps like cuts and bruises. Wear exercise sandals instead. They'll keep your feet safe, and help the circulation.

A General Thought

As we get older it's a good idea to see a chiropodist at least once a year. Only use a chiropodist who is state registered. That means they've done a three-year degree course in feet and really know what they're talking about, so you can be sure your feet are in good hands.

If your feet are in good condition, a visit will help keep them that way. If you have problems, then a session can bring about almost instant relief. Investing a small amount of time pays dividends immediately, and keeps you mobile. You really will feel you're walking on air.

Reflexology

I love having my feet massaged. It's soothing, and an instant relaxer. So I'm a natural convert to reflexology.

It works on the principle that nerve endings in the feet are connected to every single organ, gland and muscle group in the body – a sort of route map of your entire system. By massaging and stimulating different parts of the feet, you can ease many of the problems and symptoms that affect other areas by encouraging the body's natural ability to heal itself. For instance, the soles of the feet are connected to the heart and lungs, the instep to the stomach and liver, while the sides of the feet have an effect on the small intestine and bladder, and the toes release pressure in the sinuses, and so on.

My own reflexologist, Tony Porter, tells me he's able to identify subtle changes in the texture of the feet when he finds a problem area. That's when it starts to hurt. Releasing the tensions and toxins in the system means working away at the problem area until it's clear. But it's worth the short-term discomfort. The therapy can bring relief to a range of problems from headaches and blocked sinuses, to digestive disorders, gynaecological ailments, muscular pain and poor circulation.

It's especially effective as we (and our feet) get older, in boosting circulation and providing non-invasive relief to the whole system.

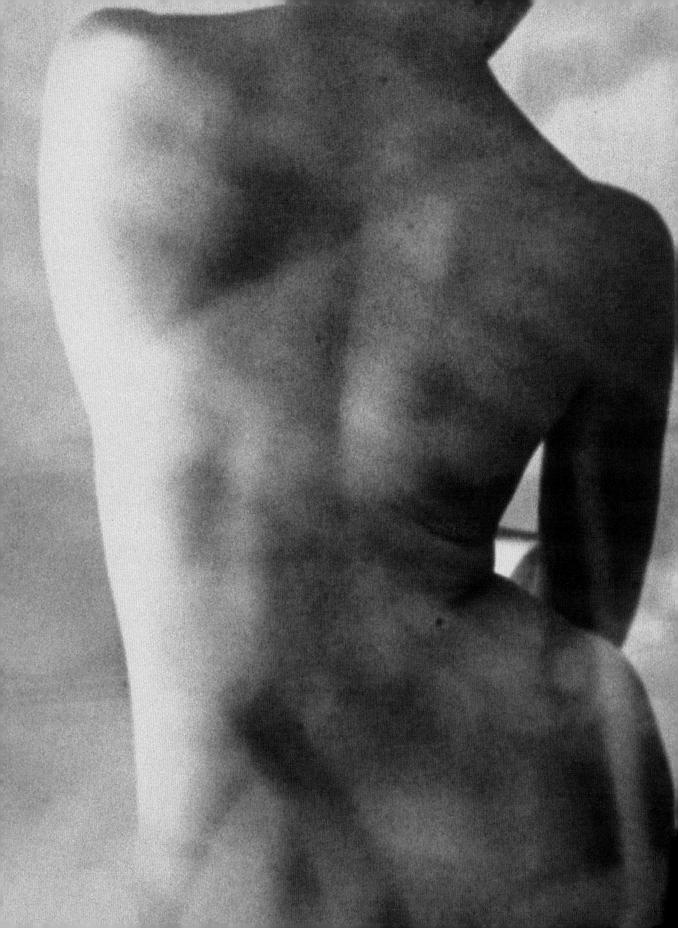

9 COSMETIC SURGERY

Not so many years ago having a facelift was something you did in secret, possibly abroad, hoping that as few people as possible would be aware of your vanity and self-indulgence. Once the bandages came off and the scars were healed, if people noticed anything at all, you just smiled politely, thanked them for the compliment, and quickly changed the subject. Boy, have times changed. According to a leading cosmetic surgery group, more than 100,000 Britons paid for cosmetic surgery during 2002 – and the numbers are rising annually.

Women (and increasingly men) now proudly discuss their cosmetic procedures in newspapers, magazines and on television, allowing us all to share in the 'before and after', as well as the often bloody and painful during. Prices have come down, techniques have improved and there's no longer any social stigma or disapproval attached to letting a surgeon roll back the years or improve your looks after years of neglect.

What's interesting is that many surgeons are now just as keen to promote anti-ageing procedures that keep you away from the knife for as long as possible, rather than suggesting surgery as a first option.

COSMETIC SURGERY

The Non-Surgical Route

Dai Davies is one of this country's top reconstructive and cosmetic surgeons, and the man I trust more than any other when it comes to getting advice on cosmetic surgery. As well as performing surgical solutions, he and his partners at their hospital in West London also run a programme called Renascence, during which they examine a patient's entire lifestyle and recommend changes that will help improve the quality of their skin and their looks in general. 'There is no point in doing a facelift on a person who smokes and spends their life in the sun,' Dai Davies says. 'Both those things cause more damage to the skin than anything, so the effects of a facelift will be very short-lived.' Instead, they discuss a programme of skin care and diet, and suggest non-surgical options that might include Botox, fat injections or fillers. If you're considering going down that route, this is what you need to know about the main methods used.

It's fashionable for some women to throw Botox parties where a practitioner offers all sorts of non-surgical remedies during a girls' gathering in the comfort of your own home. Be very careful. These treatments should only be considered when you've had plenty of expert advice, and time to think about them. Never undertake any form of treatment as the result of peer pressure, or after too many social drinks.

Botox

Botox is a chemical toxin, botulinum toxin, which has the ability to freeze muscles when injected, using a very fine needle, into the brow area, or at the sides of the eyes and in some cases in the neck. It temporarily blocks the muscles in those areas, preventing excessive movement and leaving you with a smooth, line-free complexion for up to three months.

The treatment takes only minutes, though the total consultation should last about half an hour. Go to an expert, such as a surgeon who understands the muscular structure of the face, or there could be complications like droopy eyelids. Even though the material is a toxin, don't worry. According to Nick Percival, one of the leading experts on Botox for both medical and cosmetic use, 'You will only be injected with about 100 units of Botox. You would need to ingest 3,000 to 10,000 units before registering any medical reaction. Over time, the body's own immune defence system totally clears the Botox from your body, so there is no cumulative effect from repeated treatments.'

Average cost £250 for one area.

Fat Injections

Fat is sucked from another part of your body, usually the thighs or hips, and injected into your face to fill out areas that are lined or sagging. Because it's material from your own body there should be no adverse reaction or rejection.

French surgeon Jean Louis Sebagh thinks this is the best way of improving the looks of a woman whose face is gaunt and lined. He says that doing a 'drag and lift' facelift on some thin, mature faces is a complete waste of time, and ends up looking too false and stretched. He believes in giving a woman's face volume, to make it look rounder and younger.

Average cost £3,000.

Fillers

These are injections containing hyaluronic acid, which occurs naturally in the skin, to keep it plump and hydrated. It's the loss of this substance that contributes towards the skin wrinkling and showing signs of age. The gel will fill out fine lines and wrinkles, give volume to the face and last up to nine months. Check on the ingredients in the filler your surgeon uses. Some are made from cockerels' beaks, so if you have an allergy to eggs or chickens, stay well clear. Ask for one that is free from animal extracts – there are several. As I write this, there are fifty-six different fillers available; some give permanent results, others temporary ones. Check exactly what you're being given before treatment. If you go for a permanent filler and don't like the result – you're stuck with it.

Average cost £220 per ampoule.

Collagen

Collagen is found naturally in the skin, giving it tone and suppleness. We lose collagen through a combination of ageing, muscle activity and environmental damage. The replacement collagen is derived mainly from cows, and sometimes pigs. Once injected, it will plump up the skin, with the effect lasting about four months. A consultant will want to do a skin test on your forearm to check for any allergic response before giving you the treatment, and it can take up to four weeks to get the results back before you have the treatment.

Average cost £300

The Surgical Route

Opting for cosmetic surgery is a very personal decision, one that only you can make for yourself. Remember that many procedures require a general anaesthetic and can involve considerable pain or discomfort, so be under no illusions that these are quick and easy fixes. But, in the hands of an expert, you can wipe years off your face and body.

Facelift

If you've ever stood in front of a mirror, put your hands on either side of your face and pulled your skin back, then you have some idea of how your face might look after a facelift. No more sag, no more droop, and most of the lines smoothed away, leaving your face looking like it did ten or fifteen years earlier.

There's a whole range of things a surgeon can do to lift your face and neck back into shape. They can get rid of the long lines on either side of your nose, take away the excess fat and skin that make ageing droops and folds over your bones, tighten up your jawline and even get rid of the 'turkey neck' that affects so many women in later years.

Immediate after-effects This is major surgery and will be done under general anaesthetic needing at least one if not two nights in hospital. Pain levels will be quite high for several weeks, and the swelling can take anything up to six months to disappear completely, depending on the level of surgery you've undertaken.

Effect A whole new, younger you.

Average cost From £3,850 to £9,000 if you've gone for the whole works with an eye and brow lift at the same time.

Brow Lift

As facial muscles get weaker with age, eyebrows gradually start to droop, causing excess skin to collect in folds above the eyelids. Very often a brow lift is all you need to open up your eyes, rather than surgery on the lid itself. Using keyhole surgery, a small incision is made behind the hairline and the muscle close to the nose that pulls the brow down is weakened. The skin is then gently pulled back up to reposition the arch of the eyebrow. Carried out under general anaesthetic; it should not need a night in hospital.

Immediate after-effects Noticeable bruising from the eye area to the cheeks; there may be some numbness and limited movement in the forehead. Normal sensations should return within a week, with all signs of surgery gone in three weeks. Hair regrowth around the incisions takes about three months.

Effect Eyes looking younger and less tired.

Average cost £4,000.

There is a range of options for cosmetic surgery to the face. But before committing to any procedure, be sure to follow the checklist starting on page 139.

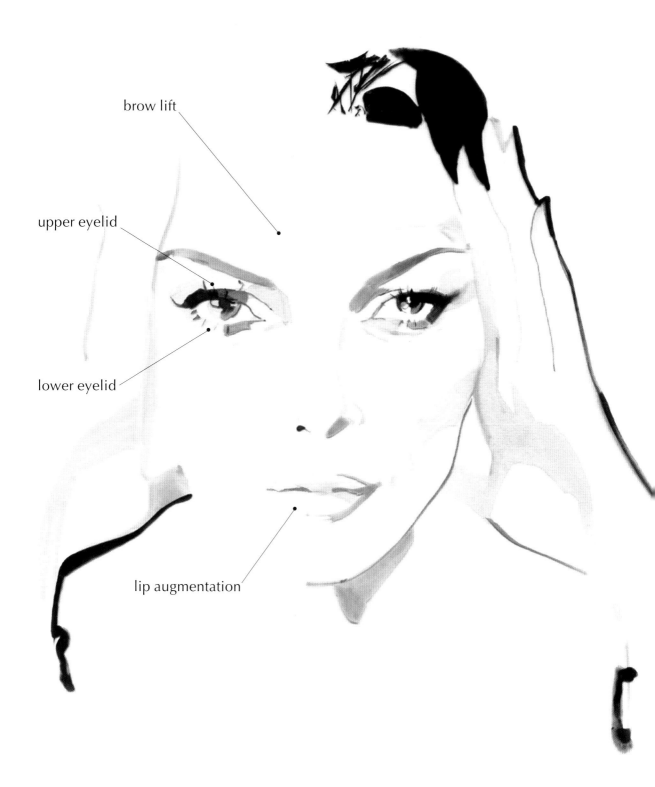

brow lift

upper eyelid

lower eyelid

lip augmentation

Upper Eyelid

A long, elliptical cut is made along the upper eyelid crease towards the crow's feet, to remove excess fat and skin. The operation is done as a day case under local anaesthetic.

Immediate after-effects Swelling and bruising for about ten days. Stitches removed three to five days after the operation. Scars must be protected from strong sunlight for several months. Loss of sensation in the lids for about six weeks.

Effect More fresh faced and wide awake.

Average cost £1,700.

Lower Eyelid

Getting rid of the bags under the eyes means cutting just below the lower lash line or inside the eyelid, teasing out the excess accumulated fat, and 'draping' the skin, rather than over-tightening it, back into place. Done under local anaesthetic as a day case.

Immediate after-effects Bruising and general puffiness for at least two weeks. Stitches removed after five days.

Effect Eyes that look at least ten years younger.

Average cost £1,700.

Both the upper and lower lids can be done at the same time, but that would usually mean a general anaesthetic and a night in hospital.

Average cost £3,520.

Lip Augmentation

A sliver of skin and fat is removed from either the tummy or buttocks, and slid into a tunnel in the lips. It will leave a small scar, but this can always be covered with lipstick.

Immediate after-effects Swelling and bruising of the lips for a few days; two to six weeks before all signs of surgery disappear.

Effect Fuller lips that will last longer than either collagen or Gortex implants.

Average cost £2,500.

Mastopexy

Quite simply perking up the breasts. Gravity, poor muscle tone and the after-effects of childbirth can all contribute to droopy breasts. They can be lifted to give you a much more youthful figure and cleavage.

Immediate after-effects Twelve weeks before signs of surgery disappear.

Effect A firm, attractive bust line.

Average cost £4,000.

Breast Reduction

Page three girls may love them, but most of my friends who have large busts find them a constant source of aggravation and discomfort. They all complain of not being able to find really nice underwear, and never finding clothes that fit and look good on them: they hate the fact that their bra straps are constantly digging into their shoulders, that they can't run or exercise without the discomfort of 'boob bounce', and that the weight of their busts drags them forwards and affects their posture.

Broadcaster Katie Boyle was given a breast reduction operation as a birthday present from her much loved late husband some years ago. I remember her telling me she felt 'liberated' after years of being imprisoned by her boobs.

Immediate after-effects You'll need to spend one or two nights in hospital, and avoid all unnecessary activity in the arms and shoulders during two to three weeks' convalescence. It will take up to twelve weeks before the signs of surgery disappear.

Effect Throw away your old bras, and enjoy your new slimline figure.

Average cost £5,000.

Breast Implants

By the time most women reach fifty they're usually pretty comfortable with the size and shape of their breasts. But some may suddenly get a rush of blood to the head and decide they need 'a boob job'. My advice is: don't. The operation sounds pretty straightforward: a surgeon inserts a sack of silicone into each of your breasts to reduce sag and increase size, but working on *Healthcheck*, one of the BBC's medical programmes, for five years, I've seen the other side of the operation. I've met women who have appalling running sores on their breasts, and who are so ill and weak that normal life has ceased and they've become housebound invalids. In each case, they were convinced that leakage from the silicone was responsible for their condition. Certainly, some of the medical evidence I've seen of horrific ulcers and open wounds on breasts would be enough to put you off for life.

As a result of the work I did on the programme with my producer Maria Polhoska, the government agreed to a year-long moratorium on breast implants for all but purely medical needs while they looked into the problems. Women who had undergone mastectomies were still offered augmentation using saline sacks rather than silicone. The ban has been lifted now, but there are stricter regulations in place to protect women's health and ensure the safety of implants. Breast-cancer sufferers still have every opportunity to undergo the safest of surgical implants, but when it comes to satisfying vanity – sorry, I can't go there. I'd recommend you improve your posture, drop your shoulders, throw out your chest and get a good padded bra.

Arm Reduction

The best way to improve skin tone and firm up flabby underarms is to exercise (see Chapter Thirteen). However, if you have 'batwings' of flesh hanging from your arms, it is possible to remove them surgically, but be warned: not many surgeons like doing this, as it's impossible to avoid having a long scar running the length of the arm from armpit to elbow.

Immediate after-effects Some discomfort, and three to six months before the area settles down.

Effect No more flabby bits, but a permanent scar.

Average cost £3,500.

Abdomen Reduction

Because women naturally store fat on their thighs and tummies, this is an area that can stubbornly resist all exercise and diet, and still give you a pot belly. Liposuction is an instant way to clear your stomach, hips and waist of unwanted fat and where excess flesh is left behind, a tummy tuck will complete the 'flattening' process. It's painful and expensive, but it works, which is why it's become the most common cosmetic procedure in the West. This is what happens: under general anaesthetic the surgeon makes a small incision in the skin and inserts a stainless-steel tube into the fatty tissue. Fat is then sucked out, rather like a vacuum might suck up dirt or water. Once you come round from the anaesthetic you'll feel as though you've gone ten rounds with Mike Tyson because the bruising can be quite extensive. You'll have to wear a surgical corset, to hold everything in place, for about six weeks. After that you'll have a nice fat-free tummy – until you overeat and cause the cells to fill up with fat again.

Immediate after-effects Considerable discomfort. You will be in hospital overnight after a general anaesthetic; stitches will be removed after twelve days; and it will be three to six months before all signs of surgery disappear.

Effect A nice flat tummy. The results can be dramatic, and very satisfying.

Cost Between £2,500 and £4,000, depending on the extent of the surgery.

Face Peel

This is a way of stripping the face of tired old skin, fine lines and some light scars. There are two methods. First, dermabrasion, which can be compared with sandpapering. Second, peeling, which is more like using paintstripper. Both methods take away the horny outer layer of skin (the epidermis) and part of the dermis below. Both promote the production of natural collagen and encourage the skin to reconstruct itself with a fresher healthier surface and fewer lines. It will not have any effect on sagging or droopy skin or the main furrows on either side of the nose.

Immediate after-effects Considerable pain! With dermabrasion there will be bleeding and the skin will be painful and swollen for a week. A scab will develop after a couple of days and lift off in seven to ten days. Peeling will produce a similar result, though not so intense, but it will be several days before you want to face the world, and three to six weeks before the skin returns to normal.

Effect Fresher, younger-looking skin.

Average cost From £900 to £1,300.

Checklist

Here is a checklist of things to consider and do before going anywhere near a surgeon's knife:

* *Be sure of your own motives* for wanting cosmetic surgery. Perhaps you're healthy and active and think your appearance no longer matches the way you feel about yourself, or maybe you don't mind the lines on your face, but can't stand the droopy skin hanging off your neck which prevents you wearing the clothes you want. Whatever the reasons, discuss them with your surgeon and be realistic about your expectations. By all means anticipate the way you will look after the surgery, but remember that while the knife can eliminate most lines and reduce fat, what it can't do is eliminate the old you and reduce your problems. You may have a new face, but you won't be a new person.

* *Become an expert* on the treatment you are considering. Talk to friends who've had similar treatments. Read books, articles, web pages, whatever you can find that will give you all the information you need about the procedures. The more knowledge you have, the better equipped you'll be to ask the right questions and make sure you're getting exactly what you want from someone really qualified to do the operation.

* *Always plan to see two surgeons* before deciding on the individual who will perform any operation so you are able to make an informed choice, and not be flattered or rushed into making a decision.

* *Ask the surgeon what experience they've had* in the operation you're considering. You need to know if they do two of these operations a year, or twenty. You want a specialist, someone who really knows what they're doing, not someone who just

pops in from time to time to knock off the odd facelift to pay for a trip to the Caribbean.

- *Ask where the surgeon trained and what their background is*. A fully trained surgeon will be on the specialist register of the General Medical Council. The initials FRCS (Fellow of the Royal College of Surgeons) on their own mean nothing in the context of cosmetic surgery. Ideally, you want someone who is a consultant plastic surgeon, though some ophthalmic surgeons have become experts at performing cosmetic surgery around the eyes, while ear, nose and throat specialists, as you'd expect, are often highly adept at performing cosmetic work on ears and noses. Surgeons in other specialities rarely have the experience to work successfully on cosmetic transformations.

- *Your surgeon should have done time in the National Health Service*. That way you can be sure their training has been recognized, assessed and validated.

- *If dealing with a foreign surgeon, ask why they're working in Britain* and not in their home country.

- *Check out follow-up provisions*. If the surgeon travels constantly between Britain and other countries (Europe and America for instance) ask what happens if there are complications after your operation and they are not in the country. Similarly, if you decide to go on a 'surgical safari' to another country, check out what happens if there are complications once you get home.

- Look at the staff in the consulting rooms, and notice the way you're dealt with on the telephone. *The whole team should be as professional and caring as the surgeon*.

- *Ask about the hospital* in which the operation will be performed, *and who the surgeon intends to use as an anaesthetist*.

- *Look carefully at the literature in the consulting rooms*, and the way the surgeon presents the before and after examples of his work. You can gain a lot by seeing exactly how he has performed on other patients in the past.

- *If you feel you are being bullied or pressured* into a decision, take a deep breath, say, 'Thank you very much,' and *leave*.

- *Price should be very low on your list of priorities*. It's the level of care and expertise and the quality of the finished product that should help you make your choice. Going for the cheapest option should not be your primary consideration. Believe me, I've seen too many examples of women whose faces have been ruined by so called 'surgeons' who offered a cheap operation that ended in disaster.

- *Once you've gone through every question with the consultant, leave and think.*
  If there is even the slightest niggle of doubt or unhappiness, visit surgeon number two and only then make a final decision.

One final thought. No one undertakes cosmetic surgery lightly, but if it makes you feel good – go for it, and enjoy the new, younger-looking you.

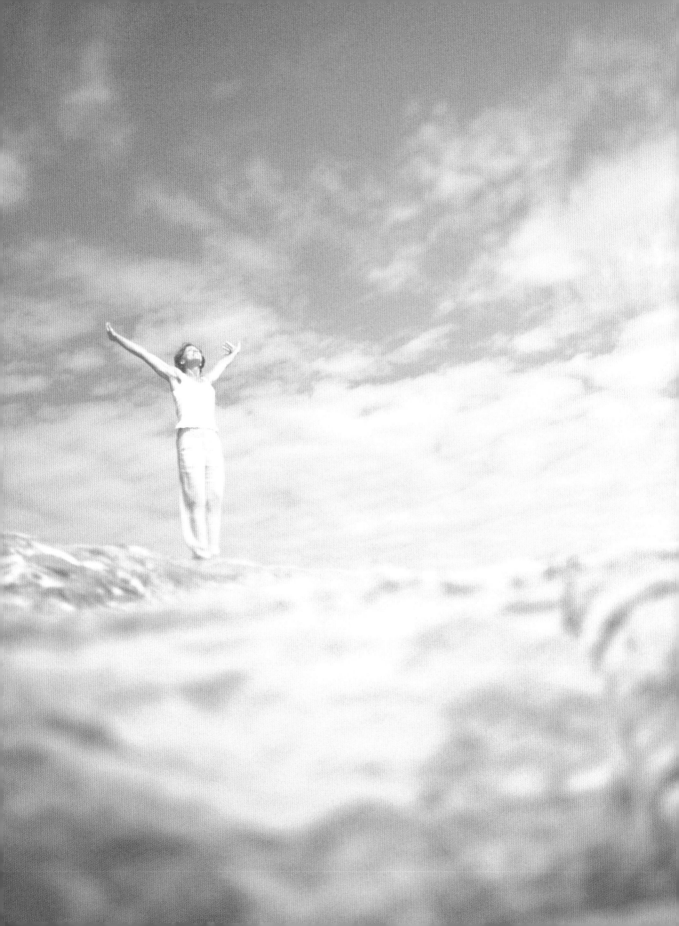

10
MENOPAUSE

Over the past few years it's true to say that the one subject that's dominated my post bag has been the menopause and hormone replacement therapy (HRT).

Scores of women who are approaching the menopause, are in the middle of it, or who have survived and come out at the other end, still have so many questions and anxieties about how to deal with the symptoms of the menopause and the long-term effects of taking HRT.

Well, I don't pretend to be an expert. What I am is a journalist who's had the opportunity of researching the subject in some depth for a range of articles and television programmes. But perhaps more importantly, I'm a woman in my fifties which means I've been there, done that, and had the hot flushes as well as the T-shirt. So my advice when writing back to women or chairing discussions on the subject is always based on personal experience laced with some pretty comprehensive background research and overlaid with more than a dash of common sense.

MENOPAUSE

Recognizing the Symptoms

Like all women of fifty or thereabouts, I recognized that, like menstruation, the menopause is something we just can't avoid. It's part and parcel of the wonderful genetic cocktail that makes us women. Swimming around in that cocktail for most of our lives is a rich and natural supply of oestrogen which is what makes us fertile during the child-bearing years, helps to keep our bones strong and our skin plump and supple, as well as providing a natural defence against heart disease. Once our bodies decide we don't need to produce eggs any more, then the oestrogen starts to run out as well, and that's when we not only start to lose some of those natural defences, we also begin to experience a chain reaction of complicated hormonal changes. As we know, those changes produce a whole range of physical and psychological symptoms ranging from the mild to the downright uncomfortable and, in some cases, to serious character-altering complications. As one of my male colleagues put it, 'My mother was always the gentlest, most reasonable woman alive, then suddenly, with the menopause, she turned into Beelzebub.' Recognize the description? Fortunately not everyone reacts in that way, and even if you do, it doesn't last for ever. Once our hormones settle down again, life gets pretty much back to normal. But in the meantime, we have to make things as comfortable as possible for ourselves (and everyone else!) by dealing with the transition and managing the symptoms.

Keep a canister of mineral-water spray in the fridge (Evian and Vittel both make them). If you get a hot flush while you're cooking, doing the housework, or have guests, a quick spray will cool you down, and the mist is so fine it will dry quickly, and even help to hydrate your skin!

Most Common Symptoms of the Menopause
Hot Flushes and Night Sweats

During the menopause, a woman's natural temperature-control system can malfunction so the body stops controlling body heat. Result – hot flushes which can occur at any time, night or day, and affect about 70 per cent of menopausal women to a greater or lesser extent. During the day they may cause a certain amount of discomfort and, for some women, acute embarrassment. At night they can disturb sleep patterns which may lead to insomnia, irritability and difficulties with memory and concentration.

Vaginal Dryness
A lowering of the body's natural oestrogen levels robs the vagina of its natural lubricant. This can make intercourse uncomfortable, even painful. It's quite natural for some women (and men!) to lose interest in sex as they get older, but for women of fifty plus the loss of libido can be aggravated by a combination of menopausal symptoms. What with all those uncomfortable sweaty nights, disturbed sleep patterns, possibly a bit of depression and vaginal dryness, is it any wonder that sex becomes less exciting? Vaginal lubricants will help, but equally important is talking it through with your partner. If he understands the problems you're having, he is more likely to be supportive, so that together you can avoid any major conflicts or difficulties in your relationship. Remember, managing your emotions and personal relationships is all part of managing the menopause.

Urinary Problems
To be technical for a moment, what can happen is that the tube carrying urine out of the bladder (the urethra) starts to work less well. This can lead to an urgent, or uncontrollable, need to pass water. You may find that you have to go to the toilet more often, and might even occasionally experience pain or difficulty while passing water. You could even begin to notice mild incontinence or leaking. Pelvic floor exercises will help (see page 204).

Psychological Symptoms.
These can include mood swings, depression, anxiety, irritability, tiredness and lack of energy. But don't forget that around the age of fifty there are often lots of other things going on in your life besides the menopause, which can affect your state of mind. You may find yourself responsible for, or worrying about, ageing or less independent parents or having to face up to the deaths of those who are closest to you. There may be family financial worries, job insecurity, the feeling of loneliness once the children have 'flown the nest', even sudden depression brought on by having to come to terms with growing older. Any number of things can combine to make you feel stressed or unable to cope, not simply those irritating menopausal symptoms. No two women are going to react the

same, but if things do start getting on top of you talk to your doctor, your partner or your friends. Don't ever feel isolated and alone. All women over fifty experience the same thing – you'll get through it too, with a little help from your friends!

Hormone Replacement Therapy

The logical way to avoid the nuisance or discomfort of hot flushes, night sweats, mood swings, vaginal dryness, loss of libido and the rest, is to replace the oestrogen and fool your body into thinking it never went away, hence hormone 'replacement' therapy. We all know women – friends, family members and high-profile personalities – who've been on HRT for years and see it as the elixir of youth, refusing to let it out of their lives. They feel great, look terrific and have bags of energy well into their sixties and seventies. For several years I took it myself. As I'm lactose intolerant (which just means I don't eat or drink dairy foods) my doctor was keen for me to counteract a reduction in calcium by boosting my oestrogen levels to guard against osteoporosis, and I have to admit that I felt absolutely fine. I had none of the side effects some women experience, and it meant I sailed through the menopause with hardly a hiccup in my routine.

Most of the women who write to me have genuine anxieties about the safety of HRT, fuelled by a number of reports specifically suggesting that it can increase the risk of heart attack and breast cancer. In the wake of such reports, supporters of HRT immediately rush to its defence, while the detractors hold up the information as proof positive that HRT is the devil's own brew and that 'meddling' with nature reaps its own rewards. No wonder most women are confused. So let's just try and strip away some of the hysteria.

Firstly, everyone of fifty-plus is more at risk of heart disease or a heart attack through the change of lifestyle and diet that comes from advancing years, and the fact is that the older we get the more likely we are to die of something. Secondly, at least one of the most recent reports to come out of America was seriously flawed. Researchers had been involved in a ten-year programme to gauge the effectiveness of HRT as a specific protection against heart attack. Some women on the trial were given HRT, others a placebo. After ten years they examined the women to see which group had developed the greater protection. They stopped midway through the programme because their findings suggested that, far from protecting against heart disease, HRT increased the risk. As you can imagine, this sent panic waves through menopausal women throughout Europe and many abandoned HRT overnight. I made a half-hour programme about this for ITV and discovered that not only was the HRT used in the trial not one that is prescribed in this country but, more importantly, the women on the trial had an average age of sixty-five, meaning that many of them were well into their seventies. No woman of fifty in her right mind who was experiencing the unpleasant side effects of the menopause would be prepared to embark on a ten-year programme and risk being given a placebo rather than the real thing. It meant, therefore, that the researchers had to use women of a much higher age group, whose chances of developing heart disease were naturally greater, simply because of their age. While it's true that there are some increased health risks from using HRT, you don't necessarily get the whole story in the sensational headlines.

The bottom line is that HRT can increase the risk of heart disease slightly in healthy fifty-plus women, and there is always a risk if you have a history of heart disease in the family. Equally, there is a slightly increased risk of breast cancer. But let's put it in perspective: out of every 1,000 women between fifty and seventy who are not on HRT, the chances are that forty-five of them will develop breast cancer. If women in that same age group are on HRT for five years, then the chances increase by two to forty-seven in 1,000. For heart disease the number per 1,000 increases by four. So, yes, there is an increase in risk, but it's so small that most health advisers will take an overall view of the risks in the light of your own personal medical history and weigh up the benefits against the disadvantages, because there is no doubt that HRT does help protect against osteoporosis, and in post-menopausal women that's a real bonus.

In addition, many women who have had a hysterectomy (and it's one in five by the age of fifty-five) will most probably have been prescribed HRT as part of their post-operative treatment. For a full hysterectomy (the removal of the womb and the cervix) it is usually an oestrogen-only HRT, while a partial hysterectomy may leave part of the womb lining so that a combined HRT – oestrogen and progesterone – is prescribed. Detecting signs of the onset of menopause is often quite difficult in women who've been through a hysterectomy because they don't necessarily experience the full catalogue of symptoms. But the anxieties about their exposure to HRT and the conflict of the advantages over the disadvantages are just as real.

So if you're confused about the benefits of HRT, and want to know if you should go on it, stay on it or come off it, just talk. Talk first to your doctor and get a clear picture of your state of health and the possible risks, if any, that might be involved. If your doctor prescribes a particular pill, implant, gel or patch and it doesn't agree with you, change the prescription until you find one that's right for you. Visit a menopause clinic. Most health authorities have one (though often they are not as well advertised as they should be and many women are not even aware they exist!). Your practice nurse should be able to give you the address and telephone number of the one nearest you. They're staffed by nurses who specialize in menopausal symptoms and solutions, so you'll get an expert and sympathetic hearing to help you make the right choice in managing your menopause. Talk to the Amarant Trust (see Useful Names and Addresses, page 204). They were formed in the early 1980s to promote a better understanding of the menopause and will advise on the right sort of treatment for you, whether that's HRT or an alternative. You could also contact the British Menopause Society (address on page 204). They were formed primarily as an independent scientific society for health professionals to raise awareness about the menopause and improve the treatment that menopausal women receive, but they have produced a couple of excellent booklets, in simple non-medical language, which I have found enormously helpful. And finally, talk to your friends. Their experience and support can be invaluable, and one of them may hold the key to the way you manage your menopause.

As for me, I came off HRT about four years ago. I decided that the regime I follow of sensible diet, plenty of exercise and calcium supplements was really all I needed to keep my energy levels high, my skin looking good, and my bones in good nick. And when it comes to managing the occasional 'menopausal' symptom – well, I go back to the journalist's standby of solid research.

The Alternative Approach

Our sisters in the Far East and South America don't have the word menopause in their language because they simply don't experience the huge hormone swings and physical symptoms that are common in the West. There's a growing body of opinion that suggests this is largely due to the difference in diet. In countries where women eat lots of soya products and pulses (beans, lentils, chickpeas, etc.), cases of osteoporosis are rare, and menopausal symptoms virtually unheard of. The magic ingredients are called 'isoflavones' and they occur naturally in soya products, all the pulses, and in supplements made from red clover. They contain a plant substance called phytoestrogens that have effects similar to those of oestrogen. Random tests done here and in America show that after adding isoflavones to your diet, many of the unpleasant symptoms of the menopause can be either drastically reduced, or disappear altogether. In other words, it suggests that a change in your diet regime may go some way towards helping you 'manage' the menopause, rather than allowing it to take over your life. So now I take a daily dose of isoflavones in a red clover supplement, drink soya milk and eat lots of soya products like yoghurt and desserts, and reckon I've covered all the bases.

If you prefer the idea of managing the menopause without HRT, again start by talking to your doctor. He or she can advise you on diet and, if you have severe symptoms, prescribe suitable medication. Just think of the thousands of women who can't take HRT because they've had breast cancer. They have to manage the menopause using alternative medication and good health regimes and most of them are coping just fine. One of the things you can do to help yourself includes taking exercise, especially weight-bearing exercise which helps keep your bones strong and guards against osteoporosis. Walking, dancing, aerobics and swimming all work to keep your heart healthy and your bones strong, and in some women exercise even helps to control the hot flushes (see Chapter Thirteen). Supplements like vitamin E may help counter the thinning effects of the loss of oestrogen on your skin and hair, while black cohosh and dong quai, favoured by practitioners of traditional Chinese medicine, may help to calm the flushes, mood swings and sweats.

And if none of that appeals, you could always revert to the method used by one of my girlfriends every time she had a hot flush. She'd whip out a beautiful, feminine fan and flutter it gently in front of her face. It kept her cool, and the men fascinated!

However you decide to approach the menopause, and your life after it, the important thing is to make an informed choice. Gather as much information as you can and take a pragmatic view of the risks, advantages and alternatives. It's impossible to say how long the symptoms will last. It could be anything from twelve months to three years as no two women are the same, so it's important to ensure that the route you choose is one that genuinely suits you. That may be HRT, or any one of the dozens of alternative solutions available, or even a combination of everything.

The important thing to remember is that the menopause is just a phase we have to go through, like adolescence and teenage spots. We should think of it as being something we can manage, not have to suffer, and while it's life changing, it's not life threatening. We all survive it! It marks the end of a woman's reproductive life, which in previous generations may have led women to believe that they'd reached the end of their useful lives. Perhaps subconsciously some of us still have that hang up. Well, forget it. The menopause isn't the end, it's the beginning of a whole new, opportunity filled period in your life, which is really what this book is all about. So celebrate it, make the most of it, and that way the best is yet to come!

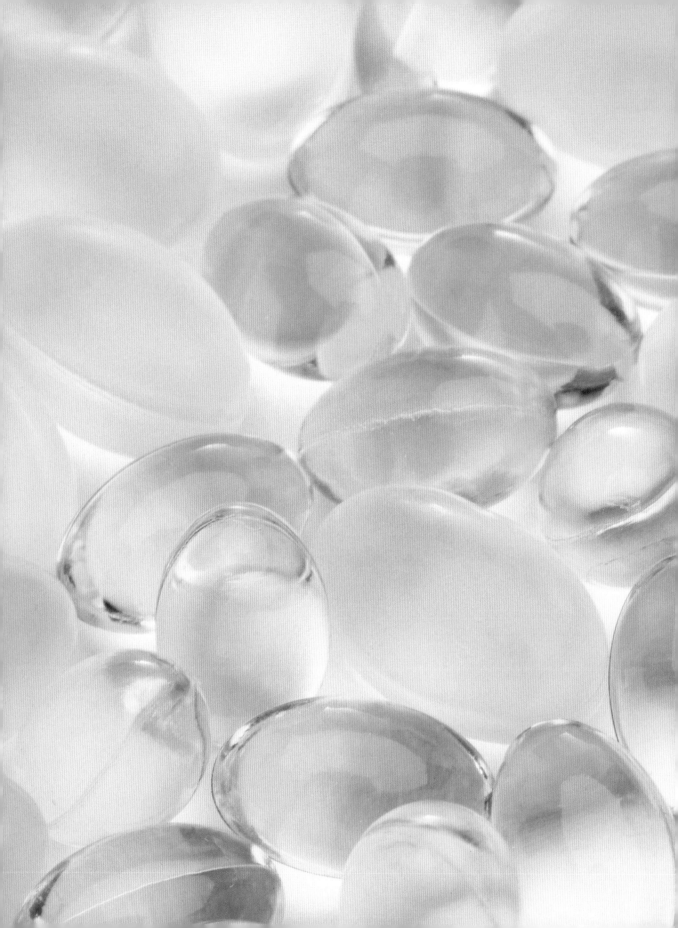

11 SUPPLEMENTS

The human body needs a cocktail of vitamins and minerals to keep it healthy and in good condition. Most people get them in sufficient quantities from a well-balanced diet or, in the case of vitamin D, from natural sunshine.

But hormonal changes and the process of ageing often deplete or rob us of these essential ingredients or system supports. Many health and beauty experts believe topping up on those supplements generally described as anti-ageing will help keep some of the ravages of time at bay. So if your system needs a little help, consult your doctor, or health-food specialist, about the supplements that could give you a boost. But don't overdose on the quantities. Take just as much as you need for a daily top-up and check with your doctor that the supplements won't react with any other medication you might be taking. Overload your system and not only could you suffer side effects, you'll also simply end up with what one of my Californian friends calls, 'Designer pee. The most expensive water in the bathroom.'

SUPPLEMENTS

Vitamin A (anti-ageing)

Important for healthy eyes and cell production, and can help resistance to certain diseases. The supplement beta-carotene is converted into vitamin A by the body, and studies have shown that people with high levels of beta-carotene are half as likely to develop a wide range of cancers from lung, to mouth, breast and bladder. It can also help in reducing the possibility of stroke.

Found naturally in Liver, cheese, eggs, butter, margarine, fish oils, and green, yellow and orange vegetables.

Recommended daily dose Women 600 mcg; men 700 mcg.

Vitamin B

Essential for the metabolism, and especially important for the elderly because a lack of vitamin B can lead to loss of memory, fatigue, irritability, insomnia and resistance to infection.

Found naturally in Liver, milk, cheese, eggs, fish, green vegetables, yeast extract, pulses, wholegrains, nuts, avocados and cereals.

Recommended daily dose Men and women 1.2–1.5 mg.

Vitamin B12

Good for healthy blood and efficient functioning of the nervous system. Can help to boost energy levels. A lack of B12 can lead to anaemia.

Found naturally in Fish, pork, eggs, cheese, brewer's yeast.

Recommended daily dose Men and women 35–40 mg.

Vitamin C (anti-ageing)

A powerful antioxidant, it helps prevent infection and repair injury. It can react with drugs such as anti-depressants and warfarin, so you must check with your doctor before taking a course of vitamin C.

Found naturally in Citrus fruits, Brussels sprouts, broccoli, strawberries, tomatoes, new potatoes and liver and kidney. The vitamin is lost if the fruit or vegetables are stored too long or overcooked.

Recommended daily dose Men and women 50 mg.

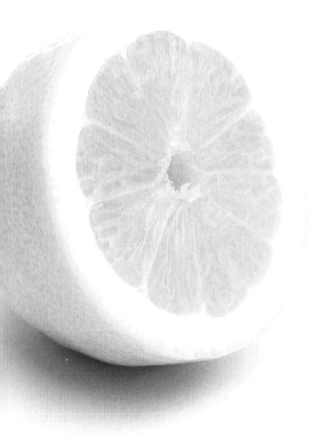

Vitamin D

Essential to help the body absorb calcium and maintain strong bones. With age, our natural levels of vitamin D drop dramatically, so it's particularly important for women over fifty to keep up a good supply of vitamin D because of the role it plays in helping to reduce the risk of osteoporosis. Research from America has shown that 50 per cent of the women being admitted to hospital with hip fractures were deficient in vitamin D.

Found naturally in Fish liver oils, vegetable and animal oils and dairy products.

Recommended daily dose Taking a supplement may not be necessary, because thirty minutes of daily exposure to sunlight (even weak winter sunlight counts) will provide the body with all the vitamin D it needs. If you do take a supplement, don't exceed 5 mcg.

Vitamin E (anti-ageing)

Another powerful antioxidant which is involved in the breakdown of fats and is especially necessary for menopausal women. It's also believed to help reduce the risk of colon and other cancers and heart disease.

Found naturally in Wheatgerm, whole grains, sunflower seeds, nuts, eggs and vegetable oils. It's destroyed by deep freezing.

Recommended daily dose 10 mg.

Multivitamins

If you can't be bothered to take vitamins individually, a single good multivitamin is an easy solution. Read the label and choose one that has at least twelve vitamins and ten minerals – then you should be covered. Check with your doctor on the maximum daily dosage in case there's a reaction to any medication you may be on.

Black Cohosh

Increasingly used as a popular remedy to help counter menopausal symptoms like hot flushes and vaginal dryness. It contains phytoestrogens, the plant compounds that have a similar effect to that of the oestrogen produced naturally by the body. Don't take black cohosh if you are on medication for hypertension as it may intensify the drug's effect of lowering blood pressure.

Recommended daily dosage 40 mg twice a day. Do not exceed this amount.

Calcium (anti-ageing)

A must for all women over fifty to help build bones and protect against osteoporosis as well as helping to prevent brittle nails. Our natural levels of calcium drop with every passing year. Do not just take calcium as part of a multivitamin. The dose you need is so high that the multivitamin will not contain sufficient to fill the daily quota.

Found naturally in Dairy foods, wholemeal bread, sesame seeds, soya products, almonds, spinach, broccoli, pulses and fish.

Recommended daily dose Women 700–800 mg; men 700–1000 mg.

Fish Oils (anti-ageing)

Fish oils, like cod liver oil, are rich in omega-3 essential fatty acids which the body needs to stay healthy. They help maintain a healthy heart and circulation, minimizing the risk of clots, and keep joints supple and flexible. The body also uses omega-3 to manufacture prostaglandins, the chemicals that regulate the activity of cells in every part of the body. Cod liver oil especially is also high in vitamins A and D.

Found naturally in Oily fish like mackerel, herring and sardines.

Recommended daily dose As directed on the label – look for one high in omega-3.

Glucosamine

Produced naturally by the body it helps to repair the damage to joints caused by osteoarthritis or injury, and is essential for maintaining healthy joints and connective tissue. As we age we produce less natural glucosamine, so a daily supplement could help boost the supply. A recent report in the *Lancet* (the magazine of the British medical profession) suggested that during a trial of the supplement, almost 50 per cent of the people on glucosamine recorded an improvement in pain levels and flexibility in their joints.

Recommended daily dose 600 mg 1–2 times a day.

Ginseng and Dong Quai

Ginseng is the herbal equivalent of testosterone (it's sometimes called the man herb). I've been taking it for years to give me energy, as it's reputed to be a great help in combating fatigue, jet lag, insomnia and nervous exhaustion. As an antioxidant it can help delay the ageing process, and can be especially useful during the menopause when stress is contributing to symptoms such as hot flushes. In China, it's used as an antidote to mental confusion and is believed to reduce the severity of Alzheimer's. Never take it with coffee (the combination of ginseng and caffeine will have you hanging from the chandelier!), and take it only for short periods of time – between six to eight weeks – then take a couple of weeks rest before starting again. It should also be avoided if you have high blood pressure.

Dong quai is considered by many to be a better tonic herb for women. It contains plant ingredients that resemble the action of oestrogens so is particularly useful during the menopause. It aids circulation, speeds tissue repair and lowers blood pressure. Not to be taken by diabetics.

Recommended daily dose Never exceed 500 mg a day.

Ginkgo Biloba

A powerful antioxidant that improves blood circulation throughout the body and brain. Because of its ability to squeeze through the narrowest blood vessels to increase supplies of oxygen to both the heart and the brain it's believed to enhance mental clarity and cognitive function. In older people, this boost is thought to improve short-term memory, and tests carried out on seniors in Australia recently showed that people on ginkgo biloba not only maintained memory function, but also carried out a series of memory tests more quickly and effortlessly than those on a placebo.

Recommended daily dose 100 mgs. Do not take if you are on blood-thinning medication.

Iron

Necessary for the formation of the haemoglobin which carries oxygen in red blood cells. It also has a role in fighting infection. A deficiency of iron leads to anaemia and can contribute to brittle nails and hair loss.

Found naturally in Liver, fish, eggs, pulses, wholemeal bread, nuts and seeds and green vegetables.

Recommended daily dose Women 10–12 mg; men 10–14 mg. **Note** excess iron is toxic and can lead to liver damage.

Selenium (anti-ageing)

Another good antioxidant, it's necessary for a healthy liver, heart and white blood cells. A deficiency is linked with an increased risk of cancer and heart disease. Some practitioners believe it can help prevent or control the onset of arthritis.

Found naturally in Brewer's yeast, sesame seeds, garlic, eggs, fish, shellfish and vegetables.

Recommended daily dose Women 45–60 mcg; men 45–75 mcg.

Finding your vitamins and minerals in natural sources and making those part of your regular diet is the best option. But from the wealth of supplements on the market you can make an informed choice for the 'extras' your body needs.

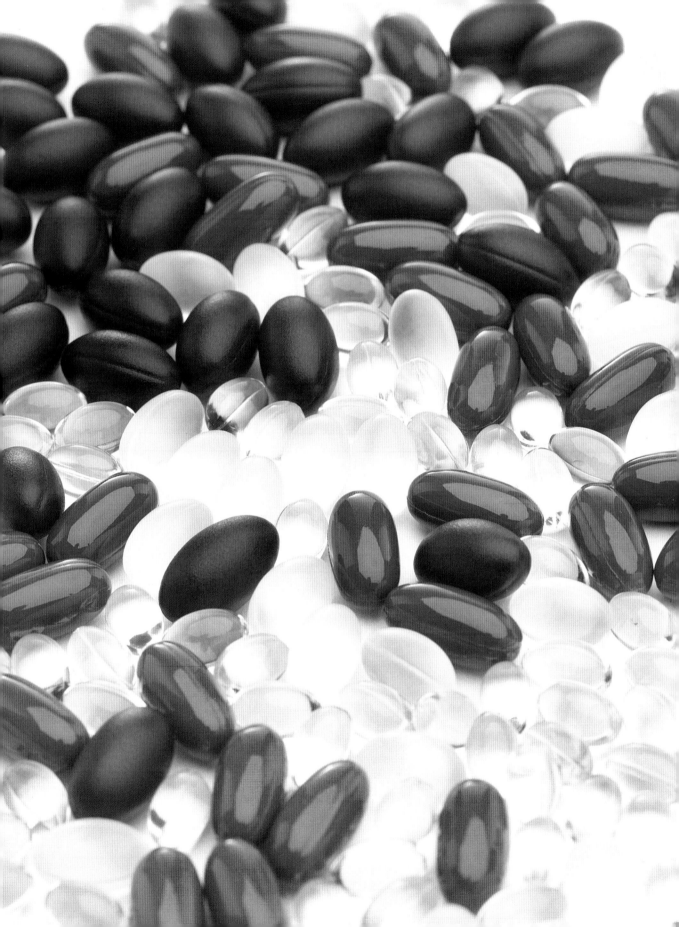

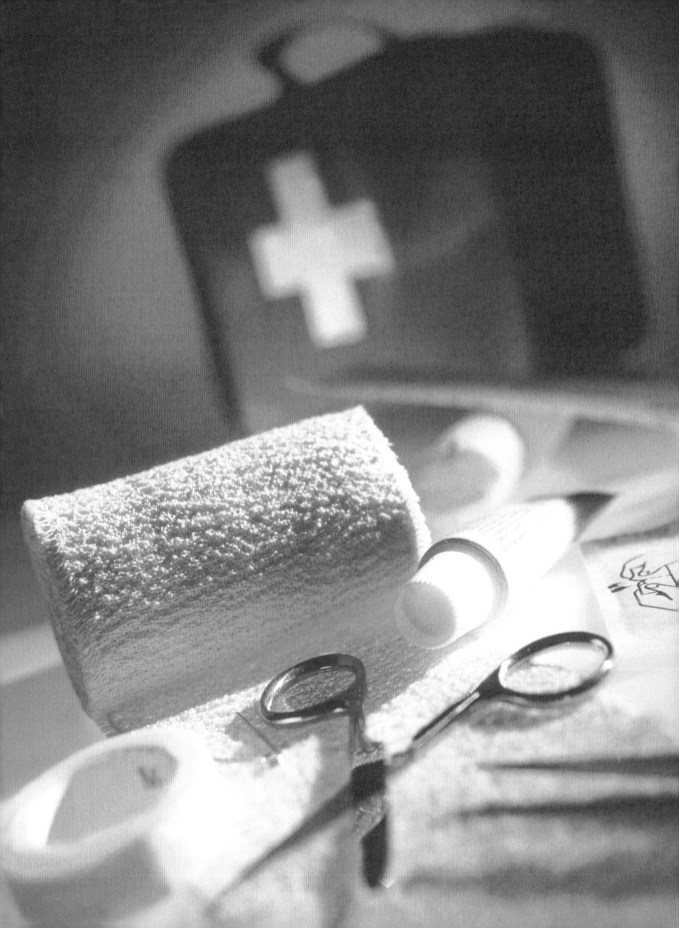

12

THINGS THAT CAN GO WRONG

When anything gets old, be it a car, a washing machine or even a favourite pair of shoes, bits start to wear out, break down and eventually fall off. Care and maintenance will keep most things going well beyond their sell-by dates, but we all have to accept that after years of constant use objects and machines become fragile and inevitably develop problems.

The human 'machine' is no different. If we keep it well oiled, well fed and in good working order, our bodies and minds will reward us with long and active service. Well, that's the theory, anyway. In the real world not everyone regularly follows a good maintenance regime, and we all at some time in our lives to a greater or lesser degree abuse our bodies. Then there's the sod's law factor of fate: something we can't escape is the fact that the older we get, the more susceptible we become to accident and illness. Yes, a healthy lifestyle can reduce the chances of you having a stroke, a heart attack, or any of the other medical problems associated with old age, but sometimes they just happen anyway.

I hope a lot of the advice contained within this book, especially the chapter on exercise, will help give you a fighting chance of being able to enjoy a long and healthy mature life. But you have to accept that sometimes things go wrong. Without trying to be a medical text book, these are some of the potential problems you need to be aware of, and guard against, as the years progress. You'll find the names, addresses and telephone numbers of specific helplines and support groups on pages 204–5.

THINGS THAT CAN GO WRONG

Memory Loss

The phrase I seem to hear being used more and more by some of my friends is, 'I'm having a senior moment,' usually after they've forgotten the name of someone they worked with for forty years, or if they can't remember why they walked into a room or what they were looking for. Sound familiar?

It really is one of the unavoidable signs of old age. Our brain cells start dying off in mid life, taking with them odd bits of memory as well as the ability to remember in general. It's not serious, just part of the body's slow and natural degenerative process though over-indulgence in alcohol will speed up the process. There are theories that suggest the brain is like one huge muscle and the more we use it, the longer it lasts. So doing crossword puzzles, or taking part in a quiz night at the local pub, could help to keep your memory and brain function sharp and responsive. I'm convinced that's one of the reasons why so many retired people watch *Countdown* on Channel 4. It's not Richard Whitley's ties that attract them, it's being able to use their brain cells! You might also want to try a course of ginkgo biloba (see page 154), which is believed to help memory function. As you approach seventy or eighty and beyond, what can happen is that the long-term memory becomes clearer while short-term memory is patchy. So it's quite possible for an eighty-year-old woman to remember the colour of the dress she wore to a party when she was five, but temporarily forget the name of her eldest granddaughter.

Once a year have a general medical check-up that includes blood pressure, pulse and urine samples. It will give your GP a fighting chance of being able to pick up any warning signs of potential changes to your general health.

The important thing to remember is that for the most part, becoming forgetful is just a straightforward symptom of old age. At best, friends and family will put it down to your age or to you being delightfully dotty. At worst, it may start to affect some of your actions or decision making, so make sure you have a good and trusted friend or adviser in your life to see you through any difficult patches.

It is not necessarily a sign of the onset of Alzheimer's.

Alzheimer's Disease

After cancer, I get the feeling that getting Alzheimer's is the biggest dread for most people of my generation, who worry about the possibility of it affecting either them or their loved ones.

Alzheimer's is not straightforward loss of memory. It's a progressive, degenerative disease of the brain that rapidly destroys brain cells, and with them the function to remember not just facts, but how to perform basic human functions. It can change a person's personality dramatically, making them aggressive or uncooperative. They may no longer be able to communicate verbally, to walk or to eat. Most distressing of all for those close to them, they may not be able to recognize their family and loved ones, and in the later stages will need twenty-four-hour care.

In spite of years of research, we are no closer to knowing exactly what causes Alzheimer's, though what we do know is that there is no conclusive genetic link within families, suggesting that it's unlikely to be inherited,

New brain-scanning technologies are leading to earlier and more specific diagnosis, but as yet there is no magic blood test or medical procedure that will identify Alzheimer's at any of its stages. Doctors and specialists have to rely on a series of tests and observations plus their skill and experience to single it out as a specific disease.

At this time there is no cure for Alzheimer's but, if detected early enough, the drugs Aricept, Exelon and Reminyl can relieve some of the symptoms, and research is going on to find a vaccine that will halt the development of the proteins which cause damage to brain cells. But even with drugs, the disease will continue to progress for anything between five and fifteen years from diagnosis.

Diabetes

In simple terms, diabetes is a common disorder of the body where there is too much sugar in the bloodstream. It occurs when the pancreas fails to produce enough insulin to turn the sugar into energy so instead it hangs around causing mischief.

Type 1 diabetes, which requires a daily insulin injection to correct the balance, usually occurs in young people under the age of forty. But once we hit mid life, then we all become prone to the possibility of developing type 2 diabetes. In fact, current research estimates that six out of every 100 people over sixty-five have type 2 diabetes. It means there are about a million mature diabetics in Britain, and possibly as many again who are not even aware they have the condition.

Maturity-onset diabetes, late-onset diabetes, non-insulin-dependent diabetes, or type 2 diabetes are all different names for the same condition which, as one of the names suggests, is not treated with a daily insulin injection. It tends to occur in mature people who are overweight and who don't get enough exercise, in individuals who have a family history of diabetes, and in people of Asian or Afro-Caribbean descent who are five times more likely to develop the symptoms than Europeans.

It's quite difficult to detect because many of the symptoms, like tiredness, going to the loo in the middle of the night, blurred vision and weight changes can often just simply be put down to old age. But your doctor can do a blood test to check your glucose levels, which will identify the problem immediately.

Treatment is through a programme of gentle exercise and diet – aiming for foods that are high in fibre, low in fat and sugar – and in some cases you have to take tablets. Only in very rare cases will it mean having insulin injections.

There's no cure for diabetes, so once you're diagnosed with type 2 you have it for the rest of your life. But it's easily managed and should not affect the quality of your life.

There are a couple of things you should be aware of: if you smoke, you should give up immediately. Diabetics have a real risk of health complications, especially heart disease. It can affect your circulation, which in turn can lead to other complications. If you are prescribed tablets for your diabetes, and are a car driver, you need to inform the Driver Vehicle Licensing Agency. If yours is a diet-only regime then you won't need to do this. But for the tablet takers you'll be issued with an 'until 70' licence. And everyone with diabetes – including those treated by diet only – should tell their motor insurance company that they have the condition.

If you like a daily tipple, the good news is that you don't have to give up alcohol, just keep to the sensible limits of a maximum two drinks per day for women and three for men. The even better news is that you can protect yourself against developing diabetes in the first place by eating a healthy, low-sugar diet, taking gentle but regular exercise and – giving up smoking!

Stroke

The human brain is an amazing example of computer engineering. It drives, commands and maintains every single cell and function in our bodies. To do this it needs a constant supply of oxygen and nutrients, so if, for some reason, that supply gets cut off, then the cells in the brain very quickly start to die of starvation or damage. That's what happens when you have a stroke.

It may occur because a blood vessel bursts inside the brain, or because the main artery leading to the brain is blocked; either way, depending on the number of brain cells damaged, the results can range from a few relatively minor, treatable conditions to paralysis and long-term disability.

The risk to women is greater than many people realize. Figures from the Stroke Association show that women have a three times greater risk of suffering a stroke than of developing breast cancer, while strokes are responsible for 15 per cent of all female deaths.

So how do we cut down the risks? Well, first of all – stop smoking (I know, this must sound like I'm nagging – but smoking really is a killer, and this won't be the last time I mention it!). Smoking doubles your risk of stroke because it furs up the arteries and makes the blood more likely to clot. So giving up smoking is one of the most important things you can do to halve your risk of having a stroke.

But the one thing you must do is avoid hypertension, or high blood pressure, because this is the single biggest risk factor for triggering a stroke. It contributes to furring up and hardening the arteries, and puts strain on the blood vessel walls, increasing the risk of a blood vessel bursting and bleeding into the brain. If you take more exercise, eat a healthy diet, reduce the amount of salt you eat, drink sensibly and watch your weight, this will all help to keep your blood pressure under control.

Symptoms to watch out for in a full stroke are a sudden numbness or weakness on one side of the body, slurred speech, blurred or lost vision, especially in one eye, and dizziness, unsteadiness or a severe headache. If you or a partner develop any of these symptoms, get medical help immediately – time is of the essence.

Sometimes people will have what's called a 'mini stroke' (proper name: transient ischaemic attack, or TIA). This happens when the brain's blood supply is only briefly interrupted. Symptoms may last for as little as twenty-four hours, and afterwards there is usually a full recovery. While not as serious as a full-blown stroke, it indicates that a part of the brain is not getting enough blood, and there is a real risk of a serious stroke occurring in the future. So *don't* ignore it, and tell your GP as soon as possible.

As with most health risks there are many things you can do to improve your chances of avoiding the problem in the first place. But if you do nothing else, you must get your blood pressure checked regularly by your GP or practice nurse because high blood pressure often has no outward symptoms and your body could secretly be harbouring a potential killer.

Heart Disease

Not a lot of people know this – but heart disease is the single biggest killer of women in this country. It claims more lives than breast cancer and stroke put together, which means 1 in 6 women will die from chronic heart disease (CHD) every year. If you thought it was a problem primarily for the men in your life – think again. In 2001, more than 54,500 women died from CHD versus 66,400 men, so there's not a lot of difference.

Symptoms to look out for as an indication that you might be having a heart attack include severe pain in the centre of the chest which may spread to the arms, neck, jaw, face, back or stomach. There might also be sweating, light-headedness, nausea or shortness of breath. Very often, women will dismiss these symptoms as indigestion, a bit of natural breathlessness or muscular discomfort, and not even recognize they are having a heart attack or the onset of angina at all. And that's the danger. Because women don't realize just how susceptible they are to CHD, the condition very often goes undetected and untreated for too long.

The causes of CHD are exactly the same for men as for women. A gradual build-up of fatty material within the coronary arteries has the same effect on your body as the plumbing clogging up in your home. The pipes get narrow, and reduce the amount of oxygen-rich blood that gets to the heart, causing the pain known as angina. In a worst-case scenario, the pipes become completely blocked – usually with a blood clot – and the heart just stops working. End result: heart attack.

Avoidance follows the well-worn path of eating a healthy diet, avoiding high blood pressure and high cholesterol, exercising regularly, keeping your weight under control, and yes – you guessed it – giving up smoking.

If there's a family history of heart disease or diabetes you have an increased risk of CHD, so you owe it to yourself, and your family, to reduce the risk.

Cancer

It may not be the biggest killer, but cancer certainly has the dubious distinction of being the one thing that strikes fear in the hearts of most people I know. There are more than 200 types of cancer and there is no single cause or single style of treatment. The only thing they have in common is the basic way in which cancer develops and spreads, and that is by cancerous cells in the body dividing and growing out of control.

It's a worrying indication of nature's ingenuity over man's determination that so far, despite years of research and millions of pounds in donations and government expenditure, the cause and, in many cases, the cure for cancer still eludes us. Some cancers are wholly and successfully treatable when caught early enough. Others are so aggressive that management is the only option. Perhaps it's the fact that it's so random and unpredictable that frightens us so much. Certainly, knowing your enemy has always helped even up the odds of the battle, but cancer can strike out of the blue, for no reason and without warning, often in spite of our best efforts to maintain a healthy lifestyle. As we manage to conquer other diseases and live longer, for those of us looking forward to a long and active retirement it's even more important to be vigilant about the possibility of developing cancer. Living longer means our bodies are going to be given extra exposure to cancer-causing chemicals and environmental damage like sunlight, which increases the risk of abnormal cell formation. With age, our immune system becomes less effective at identifying the abnormal cells and destroying them before they have the chance of developing into cancers. So it's vital to be aware of the warning signs that might suggest the beginnings of a tumour or some other abnormality, and discuss them with your doctor immediately. The sooner a cancer is diagnosed – the greater the chance of defeating it.

A checklist for healthy living

- Eat a sensible diet that includes five portions of fresh fruit and vegetables every day.
- Drink at least 1.5 litres of water a day.
- Reduce the salt in your diet to 4 g a day (just under a teaspoonful) and remember that many processed foods are full of the stuff.
- Reduce your sugar intake.
- Drink alcohol in moderation.
- Take some form of regular exercise.
- Give up smoking.

In women, the risk of breast cancer increases as we get older, so more than half the breast cancers in Britain affect women over the age of sixty-five. Perhaps because it attacks a part of our anatomy that is so quintessentially feminine, it seems to worry us more than any of the other, more aggressive cancers to which women are just as prone. But at least we can take precautions to identify breast tumours, and hopefully deal with them before they get out of control.

In Britain all women over fifty have the right to a regular mammogram as part of the government's health-screening programme. Don't ignore it. Take the test for your peace of mind, and possibly an early indication of a problem. Make self-examination part of your regular health and beauty routine. When you're applying body lotion it's so easy to slide your hands over your breasts and immediately notice any change in their shape, the sudden appearance of a lump or thickening. You will also find any swelling or lump in the armpit.

If you do find something please don't ignore it. My late, darling mother-in-law discovered a lump when she was seventy-nine. She didn't tell a soul for months. We all noticed she'd become withdrawn and was not her usual cheery self, but by the time we dragged it out of her the lump was the size of a small orange. She survived the treatment and went into remission, but suffered a level of anxiety and pain that could have been vastly reduced.

If a lump is found, and cancer diagnosed, you'll have every opportunity to discuss treatment and consequences with your doctor or surgeon. If you think people are being vague or less than honest, ask direct questions and insist on direct answers. It's your body they're dealing with, and you have the right to make an informed judgement on the situation. If you have to have the breast removed, take heart from the fact that reconstructive surgery will leave scars, but ensure you regain your feminine curves.

For men, the equivalent anxiety hovers around the prospect of prostate cancer. The prostate is the small male gland that surrounds the end of the tube that carries urine from the bladder to the penis. Most men of fifty-plus have some cancer cells lying benignly in their prostate and, on the whole, they grow so slowly that they are not a problem. But in some cases, after fifty, the cells can grow out of control and spread to other parts of the body, especially the bones. Most of my women friends agree that on the whole, men are notoriously bad at reacting to changes in their bodies, and we all know a few who can still be infuriatingly shy in discussing problems affecting such a personal part of their anatomy. There are signs that indicate possible problems with the prostate, and they should not be ignored.

Look for:

- Difficulty in passing urine.
- Passing urine more frequently than usual, especially at night.
- Pain when passing urine.
- Blood in the urine.
- Pain in the bones, which might suggest the cancer has spread.

Any of the above symptoms warrant an immediate check with your doctor. They may not be connected to cancer, but you just can't take the risk. It's possible to diagnose prostate cancer through a series of tests which might include a blood test, a biopsy, ultrasound, a rectal examination or a scan.

Just keep in mind the fact that because prostate cancer develops so slowly, the earlier you catch it the greater the chance of dealing with it successfully. So, guys, don't allow embarrassment or tardiness to put you off getting a check-up. Your health is frankly more important than your blushes.

As I've said, there are so many different cancers it's impossible to go into them all in a book like this, though I have dealt with skin cancer on pages 32–3.

The biggest cancer charity in Britain is called CancerBACUP. You'll find their address and contact number on page 205. They have a simple checklist of nine symptoms that may or may not indicate the presence of a cancerous tumour somewhere in the body.

1   A cough that lasts more than three weeks, or coughing up blood.
2   Hoarseness of the voice that lasts more than three weeks.

3   A lump that does not go away.

4   A sore that will not heal.

5   A change in the size, shape or colour of a mole or any change in the skin.

6   Blood in the bowel movements or urine.

7   Bleeding from the vagina.

8   Indigestion that does not go away or keeps coming back.

9   Unexplained weight loss.

Many of these things may have a totally different cause and have no connection with cancer at all. But you owe it to yourself and your family to check them out if they apply to you.

Osteoporosis

The curse of the post-menopausal woman. Once our oestrogen levels start to fall we lose one of our main safeguards for strong, healthy bones. Because they're tucked away inside so much flesh and muscle it's not possible for us to take them out, examine them and see how they're doing. Though if we could, we'd probably be appalled by what we see. In the worst cases of osteoporosis the bones look like a delicate tracery of lace work or the inside of a Crunchy bar when they should be solid and supportive.

The National Osteoporosis Society reckons that one in three women have osteoporosis to a greater or lesser extent, and while it may not actually make us feel ill, the impact of brittle bones on our long-term health and quality of life can be devastating. Any fall in later life has a dangerously high potential for resulting in a fracture, especially of the hips and wrists. In the elderly this can lead to long and painful hospitalization and the prospect of major hip-replacement surgery. According to a leading national doctor, who's an expert on the condition, in the worst-case scenario a fracture at the neck of the thigh bone puts elderly women in a category where they have a 20 per cent chance of dying from complications within six months. The figures are pretty alarming. There are, on average, 85,000 hip fractures every year, affecting both men and women over the age of sixty. Of these, 14,000 will die from complications or secondary infections arising from the fractures and about 30,000 elderly people a year will have their quality of life dramatically reduced because they will lose their mobility. Clearly we need to do everything possible to keep our bones healthy and strong.

HRT is still considered to be the best protection, provided you are fully aware of the slight increase in the risk of heart disease and breast cancer. There is also a new drug called Fosamax, which is available on prescription and pretty expensive at between £35 and £40 for a month's supply. But it's been shown to arrest and, in some cases, even reverse osteoporosis.

Eating soya products and taking a calcium supplement with vitamin D is helpful (see Chapter Eleven). Calcium on its own isn't much use; it needs vitamin D to be absorbed into the system. Most people can get all the vitamin D they need from half an hour's daily exposure to sunlight, but you may need to top this up with a supplement. A high strength vitamin D and calcium supplement is available on prescription from your doctor.

Exercise is essential. But is has to be a weight-bearing exercise, something like cycling, dancing, brisk walking, aerobics or tennis to really get the muscles working, because it's the action of the muscles pulling on the bones that helps to strengthen them (see Chapter Thirteen).

Obesity

Putting on a few extra pounds or going up a dress size is really not that important once you get into your mature years. After all, women are supposed to have curves and one of the freedoms that comes with maturity is the opportunity to feel comfortable with yourself and not be under pressure to be constantly chasing the perfect model girl figure. But there's comfortable and then there's fat, and then there's obese. Carrying too much weight in later life has a real knock-on effect on the state of your health, so if you want a long and healthy life you need to keep your weight down to a sensible and healthy level.

Being overweight not only puts you at severe risk of developing type 2 diabetes, but also increases the possibility of suffering congenital heart disease, or being felled by a stroke, and it puts such extreme pressure on your joints that mobility, or the lack of it, becomes a serious issue.

What's important after fifty is not so much your weight as your body mass index (BMI) which gives a good indication of the amount of excess fat you're carrying for your height and shape. There's a formula for working it out which is that you divide your weight in kilograms by your height in metres squared. So if you weigh 58 kg (9 st) and are 1.65 m (5 ft 3 in)tall that's 58 divided by 1.65 x 1.65, giving a BMI of 21.3. You should be aiming for somewhere between 19 and 25. BMI values over 30 are classified as obese.

If that's too complicated, get your doctor to work it out for you. They have charts that do it in a second. If the BMI suggests you need to loose excess fat, settle into a sensible eating plan – not a diet – and take gentle exercise. You'll shed pounds and a lot of health problems, and gain a few more years of healthy living.

Smoking

On average, every quarter of an hour in the UK three people die from a smoking-related illness including cancer, heart disease and stroke.

Smoking takes life-giving oxygen out of your system, and puts poisonous carbon monoxide in. Tobacco is connected to 90 per cent of all oral cancers; it damages the delicate membranes of the larynx, is harmful to the digestive system, causes chronic bronchitis, deposits tar in the lungs, affects the arteries of the brain and, because it makes the ovaries less effective at producing oestrogen, can increase the risk in women of developing osteoporosis. Oh yes, and every time you inhale the smoke you create thousands of wrinkle-forming free radicals which attack the collagen in the skin and impair the blood flow, producing a dull, lined, dry complexion, while unconsciously squinting from the smoke in your eyes promotes crow's feet. I rest my case.

Unhappy With Your Doctor?

The more dependent we are on our doctors as we go through life, the more important it is that we have a good 'working relationship' with them. I feel very fortunate to have a great GP – someone who gives me confidence and whose judgement I trust absolutely. Unfortunately, many people are sometimes either intimidated by their doctors, or feel they don't have the right, or the time, to question their actions or decisions.

If you find yourself in this position, contact the Patients Association (see page 205). It is a totally independent body established to guarantee the rights of patients and lobby for their protection. Its staff will talk your problems through with you in complete confidence and not only advise you on how to get the best out of a consultation with your GP, but also how to handle any problem that might be troubling you. That might include how to obtain your medical records, or get a second opinion or make a complaint. All of their booklets contain invaluable advice to ensure you and your family get good value and service from both the NHS and private health care. Their motto is, 'Listening to patients. Speaking up for change', and that's exactly what they do.

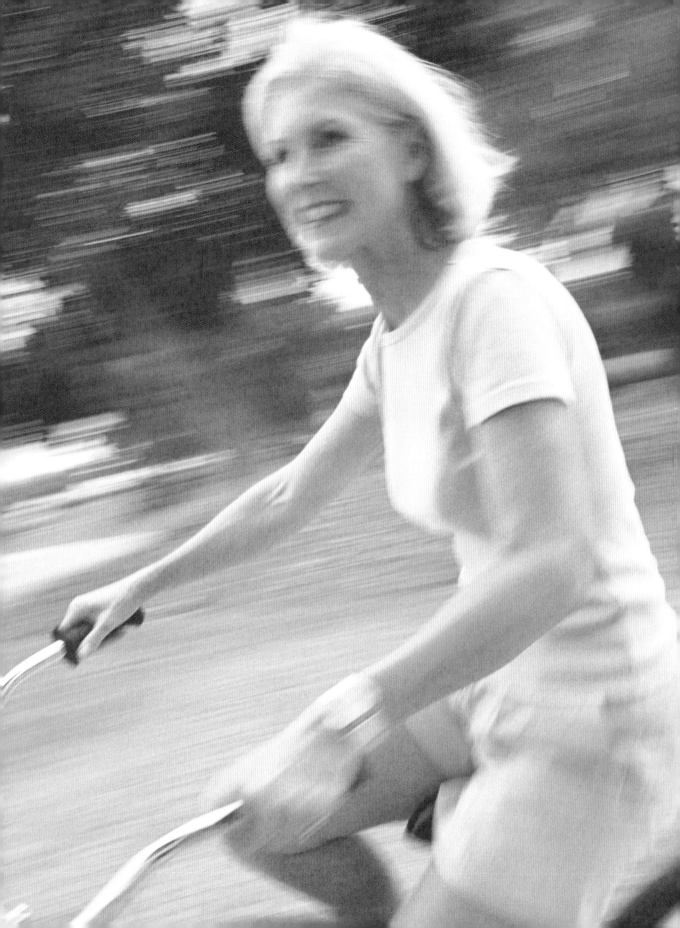

13
EXERCISE

Mention the word exercise to a lot of people over fifty and you'll see their eyes glaze over. The mere idea of doing anything that involves physical exertion, sweating, and (Lord, help us) squeezing into something Lycra is clearly both painful and anathema to them.

But the inescapable fact is that from the age of fifty to a hundred, exercise is almost more important in our lives than it was when we were thirty-somethings.

In our youth, exercise was a wonderful way of achieving and maintaining a great body shape and physical fitness, with perhaps an eye to the future in recognizing that it would help keep us healthy. From fifty onwards exercise has a wholly specific role in protecting the body against major age-related illnesses and enabling us to maintain an independent lifestyle for as long as possible. That may mean climbing Everest, or just being able to cut your own toenails and get in and out of the bath on your own. We all have our own definition of independence but whatever it is, we want to hang on to it for as long as possible.

EXERCISE
Keeping Young and Beautiful

We're lucky enough to live in a century where major medical advances have increased our lifespans beyond anything our grandparents could have imagined. Now it's up to us to ensure we make the most of that by having an increased active lifespan. I found this statistic hard to believe, but ten years ago there were just 50 people over the age of 100 in Britain; now there are 1,000, and the life expectancy graph for our generation is on a steep upwards curve. But what's the point of making it past sixty if you are so unfit that you are chair-bound and dependent on others? Frankly, there's no fun in that! Just half an hour a day, five days a week, will make a dramatic difference to your health, your mobility and your quality of life. If that sounds too much, then take it in two fifteen-minute sessions. Whatever you do doesn't have to be violent or energetic, and you don't need to become a fitness freak. You just need to do something that will make you a little breathless and a bit warmer than usual. So stay with me for the next few pages; they could make all the difference to your life.

Health Benefits

The health benefits of exercise are enormous. According to Dr Dawn Skelton of Manchester University, 'There is no medical condition, with the exception of rheumatoid arthritis during flare-up and some acute medical conditions undergoing care, that will not improve with exercise.' Exercise reduces the risk of heart disease, stroke and diabetes; by maintaining bone density you can reduce the risk of fractures from osteoporosis. It reduces the pain and stiffness in arthritic joints, brings down your blood pressure (the main culprit in promoting stroke), helps you to sleep and, even if you are bed- or chair-bound, improves the quality of your life by relieving stiffness, constipation and problems caused by poor circulation. There is even evidence to suggest that regular exercise has a beneficial effect in protecting you against forty-one separate cancers, colon cancer in particular.

Balance, Power, Strength, Flexibility, Endurance

These are the five key areas to work on to maintain a healthy life after fifty.

Balance

As babies and young children we crawl, leap and prance around in all directions without ever having to think about what we're doing. As we move into our seventies and eighties and do fewer three-dimensional activities (moving backwards and sideways as well as forwards), our brains can switch off those abilities assuming, through lack of use, they're no longer needed. It's why some elderly people become unsteady on their feet, losing their balance and falling with alarming regularity. There's a risk of serious injury and fractures, and figures from the Department of Health show that on average, only 20 per cent of patients suffering hip fractures regain total mobility.

Exercise to help your balance includes:

- T'ai chi. Imported from China, this is slow and controlled movement which gives a wonderful all-round exercise for maintaining balance, spatial awareness and coordination.
- Line dancing. Gets you moving forwards, backwards and sideways to music. Good cardiovascular exercise and, most importantly, it's fun and social.
- Ballroom dancing. All of the above, and a great way of meeting new people.

Power

Powerful muscles help ensure we maintain quick reactions. Muscles lacking power respond very slowly. So if, for instance, you find yourself tripping, or losing your balance, a powerful response from your muscles will get your arm out quickly and save you from toppling over. If you can break your fall with a quick movement you're likely to do less damage to yourself than if you hit the ground with a thump.

Strength

Strong muscles not only help build strong bones and protect against osteoporosis, they also help to support joints to relieve pain. We all need a certain amount of strength to lift and move our body weight – but we lose strength with age while often gaining some weight.

Flexibility

A third of women over fifty in Britain aren't flexible enough to be able to do up the zip on the back of a dress on their own. That may not worry you now, but as the joints stiffen and become less flexible, many of the things you do now and take for granted, like bending down to pick up something you've dropped or putting on your tights or socks, may become much more difficult and uncomfortable.

Yoga is probably the best all-round exercise regime to improve flexibility. It will lengthen and strengthen your muscles giving support to your joints, while ensuring that the joints themselves are kept mobile and flexible.

Endurance

This doesn't mean entering the marathon every year (though there are many people of seventy- and eighty-plus who do!). But research shows that a third of all people of seventy-plus can't comfortably walk a quarter of a mile on their own. They simply don't have the muscle power or lung capacity to cope without breathlessness. Regular exercise, especially walking (see page 175), will build up your endurance and stamina, improving your mobility and giving you the freedom to get out and enjoy life!

Before Starting Any Exercise

Talk to your doctor. There are real risks for people who are totally out of condition or overweight who suddenly decide to start an exercise programme. Start slowly, build up gradually and, ideally, work under the supervision of someone who knows what they're doing.

Mix and Match Your Programme

You need to do a combination of things to build your stamina and your flexibility. It's all very well being able to touch your toes, but not a lot of good if you can't walk up a flight of stairs without being exhausted by the effort. An ideal combination of exercise will boost cardiovascular strength, improve flexibility, maintain bone mass and help your blood pressure by relaxing you. So a brisk walk, or cycling to a t'ai chi or yoga class would give you the ideal combination.

Choose Something You Really Enjoy Doing

Exercise should be fun, not boring or a chore. If you hate the idea of going to a fitness class, or working through your daily half hour routine, you'll soon give it up and lose all the benefit. If it's sociable, fun to do, and makes you feel good, the psychological benefits will be as important as the physical ones. Once you find the right combination, stick to it, and make it part of your life. Once it becomes boring, swap it for another routine, but don't give up.

Things to Remember

Exercises Done on the Floor

These can produce double the benefit of exercises done standing, because we reduce the effect of gravity on our bodies. It also gives you the confidence to know you're able to get up again, provided you're not injured, if you ever take a tumble. If your floors are carpeted you should find it quite comfortable, but if they are solid and covered in tiles, wood or lino, you may want something a little softer to exercise on, like a rug or an exercise mat.

What to Wear

Be comfortable: wear loose, warm clothing or leggings, so your limbs aren't constricted and you don't get cold, or, if you are exercising in the privacy of your own home, you may prefer to work out as the ancient Greeks did – au naturel!

Medication

This can sometimes interfere with the good effects of exercise by giving a false impression of your true heartbeat, blood pressure or insulin levels. So if you are on heart pills, or taking medication for diabetes or blood pressure, check with your doctor to make sure you take your pills at the appropriate time either before or after an exercise session.

Drink Water

Do this before, during and after exercise. We all need water to counteract the effects of perspiring during exercise, but in people of fifty-plus it's especially important for two reasons. Firstly, our bodies are less efficient at controlling core body temperature, so we need water to keep us cool. Secondly, a lack of water makes our nervous system sluggish, which means we can loose coordination and get tired more quickly. When you're tired, you're more likely to make errors, and that can be dangerous.

Warm up and Stretch

You must warm up and stretch your muscles before starting any exercise session, however gentle. You can either use this warm-up or the one on page 179. Swing your arms and turn your torso to loosen up your waist. Do gentle side bends. Flex your knees and shoulders, bend forwards and (if you can) touch your toes to stretch your hamstrings. But unless you are used to doing exercise and already have a certain amount of flexibility go easy on this, and only bend as far forwards as you can. Alternatively, to stretch your hamstrings you can sit on the floor with your legs together and bend forwards, gripping your knees at first but aiming eventually to be able to grip your ankles.

Remember to Breathe

Breathe when you're exercising. Slow, regular, deep breaths will keep your blood oxygenated and your lungs pumping. When doing any lifting or strengthening work it is especially important to maintain regular breathing as these activities can increase blood pressure if the breath is held.

Listen to Your Body

Don't ever work 'through' the pain, only work 'up to it'. A certain amount of muscular discomfort or fatigue is normal when you're exercising. Pain is not. It's also normal to have some discomfort in your muscles the morning after your exercise, especially if you are new to it. Don't worry, exercise gets easier the more you do it.

Defeat Ageisim

If someone says you can't do something, or you get twinges of pain 'because of your age', don't listen to them. Giving in to ageism is the first step on the slippery slope of descending from age to disuse to disease. Reverse the equation and stay fit, stay healthy and live a longer, active life.

'Man does not cease to play because he grows old. Man grows old because he ceases to play.' GEORGE BERNARD SHAW

Getting Exercise Into Your Routine

Swimming

This is one of the best all-round exercises you can do and if you're just starting out on an exercise regime it's a good way to begin. The water supports your body and takes pressure off your joints, as well as keeping you cool so you can exercise for longer. Whether you are swimming or taking part in a water aerobics class, the movement of your body through the water will keep the muscles in your shoulders, back, legs, arms and stomach strong, lean and toned, and your whole body more flexible. It's also a terrific de-stresser. There's something about slipping effortlessly through water and being buoyed up that reduces tension, so you could find you sleep better and feel less tense during the day.

A word of caution. Many people don't like putting their head under the water and getting their hair wet. Unfortunately, if you swim, especially if you do the breast stroke, with your head poking up, you'll put undue strain on your neck and spine. Better to buy a good swimming cap, a pair of goggles, slather your hair in conditioner, and accept that you're going to have to sacrifice the hair do. Or take up water aerobics – that way you keep your head out of the water all the time, but get the full benefit of the exercise.

Walking

This has to be not just one of the best forms of aerobic activity, but also one of the easiest, cheapest and most effective exercises for people of all ages and physical conditions. I'm not talking about a gentle stroll down to the post office, or an amble out with the dog. If you're going to use walking as an exercise you have to be prepared to walk purposefully or briskly for half an hour (though if you include it as part of the dog's daily routine they'll benefit from the extra pace too!).

Make sure you wear comfortable trainers or lace-up shoes to give your ankles support and cushion the impact on your feet as you stride out. Avoid bouncing along. Instead make sure that your heel comes into contact with the ground first, and that you use the whole foot as you roll onto your toes. Swing or pump your arms as you walk. This keeps your shoulders relaxed and flexible, helps to tone the muscles on the flabby bit under your arms, and gives rhythm to your breathing and your pace.

Unlike running, walking won't jar the joints in your knees, hips and back. But it will build muscle, help to reduce the age-related loss of bone, get your heart and lungs pumping, and eventually trim down the excess weight on hips, thighs and tums. It's also another good stress-buster. If you can find a partner, or buddy to walk with you, it'll double the pleasure and give you the commitment to maintain a regular routine.

Housework

Don't ever underestimate the workout you get from vacuuming, dusting, cleaning windows and making beds. If done energetically, you'll be bending, stretching, using your shoulders, wrists and tummy muscles all to good effect. It will give you a low-impact aerobic workout, and help your flexibility and strength. But try to combine it with some other, perhaps more enjoyable, form of exercise. That way you'll be giving your body a real treat.

Cycling

A good aerobic exercise for the heart and lungs, and for maintaining bone density in the lower limbs. With city traffic it can be dangerous and you'll probably breathe in more pollutants than fresh air. But if you can cycle in a park, or in the country, you should get all the benefits and none of the disadvantages.

T'ai Chi

This was developed in China and has kept that nation fit for over 2,000 years. Offices and factories encourage workers to begin their day with a t'ai chi session, and you'll often see people, many of them in their seventies and eighties, doing it together in the parks and open spaces of China's main cities. It's sometimes described as 'meditation in motion' and can look like a very tranquil, graceful dance. It relaxes the body and the mind, helps to tone muscles with its slow, controlled movements, and is excellent for improving balance and spatial awareness.

When exercising or walking out of doors always remember to wear a sun protection cream of at least SPF15 to protect your skin from the harmful rays of the sun. Don't wear a total sunblock though – vitamin D is absorbed through the skin when we are outdoors in daylight and this is good for our bones as it enables our bodies to make calcium.

Pilates

Developed by the German physical trainer Joseph Pilates, it offers the body a complete and thorough workout. It contains elements of yoga, weight training, martial arts and even circus training. The combination of controlled exercises, many of them done on the floor, maintains strength, balance, flexibility and coordination, without putting any strain on the joints. Pilates is especially good at maintaining your posture muscles.

Yoga

Opens out the body, helping to make your muscles lean
and strong, and your whole body more supple. The level
of concentration needed will clear your mind and help relax
you emotionally as well as physically. You can learn yoga from
a book or a video tape, but a good teacher will ensure you're
performing each movement correctly and getting the
maximum benefit from each position. It's an excellent
discipline for all ages and all levels of fitness and suppleness.
But it's not a weight-bearing exercise. So to cover all bases,
a brisk walk to the yoga class will ensure your muscles aren't
just lengthened, strengthened and toned, they'll be working
on your bones to keep them healthy too.

The glorious Sophia Loren has this tip for getting in and out of chairs in a way that doesn't betray your age. Bring your bottom to the edge of the seat. Plant your feet firmly just behind your knees to give you strong leverage, place one hand on the arm of the chair or beside you on the seat, and gently push yourself up until you are standing straight and tall. If you grunt and groan and make a meal of hauling yourself out of a chair it's an instant give-away to your age and lack of fitness.

Stand Up For Yourself

Good posture can often help eliminate some of the problems people have with their
back, hips, spine and digestion. Over a lifetime, it's easy to find yourself slumping forwards,
but if you can stand up straight comfortably you'll not only look better, it will also help
your breathing, and make it easier for your body to get the maximum benefit from your
healthy diet and exercise regime. It's also the quickest way I know to 'lose' a few kilos.
Once everything is pulled in and stretched up you actually do look thinner!

Try this: clench your buttocks, tilt your pelvis slightly forwards, pull in the tummy,
raise the ribcage, relax and drop your shoulders, and put your chin up. Imagine there
is someone above you pulling a strand of your hair from the top of your head towards
the ceiling. Feel your neck get longer. Don't tense up; keep your body relaxed. If you
can maintain that posture during the day while standing, sitting or walking, you'll look
so much better (and younger!). Your spine will be realigned and you'll have taken out
any of the kinks and stresses that shouldn't be there. Take a deep breath and feel how
much oxygen you can get into your lungs – now slump and try to take in a deep breath.
Difficult, isn't it?

MY HOME WORKOUT

The great advantage of exercising at home is that you can choose when, where, how often and how vigorously you follow a routine. In the 1980s I produced a fitness tape called *Shape Up and Dance* that had a whole exercise routine set to some of the top pop music tunes of the day. Believe it or not, twenty years on I'm still getting requests for the same tape. Which means, I guess, that it must work! So I've adapted some of the exercises, and added a few extras to give you a good low-impact cardiovascular workout, improve your flexibility and strength, and tone the muscles in a few potentially problematic areas.

If you are reasonably fit, there's nothing too complicated or taxing here. But if you haven't done much exercise in the past, before embarking on this routine, read through the exercises carefully, look at the pictures and choose the easiest options with the lower repetitions. Some of the exercises are a bit advanced for complete beginners, so don't think you have to throw yourself into the routine without carefully considering those movements that will suit your body and your fitness level. Work up to the full routine gradually – there's no rush. And remember to always check with your doctor before embarking on any fitness regime.

Mix and match the exercises to suit your own needs and fitness level. Even though I have given the minimum number of repetitions for each exercise, as you grow stronger and more flexible you may want to increase the number of times you do a particular exercise to a point where you still feel comfortable and that matches your improved fitness. But don't ever overdo it.

In fact, when you're exercising on your own, it's even more important for you to follow a few golden rules to ensure you don't either overindulge or risk injury.

- Always warm up before you begin.
- Work in a room that is warm and airy, but not hot and stuffy.
- Wear loose-fitting, comfortable clothes that don't inhibit your movements.
- Drink water before, during and after exercise.
- Never do anything that causes pain, and never work through pain.
- It's normal for muscles to feel a bit stiff or achy after a workout, especially if you have not exercised for a while. A few aches are acceptable, pain is not.
- Listen to your body.
- Find an album that has a collection of music with a good, steady beat (not too frantic!) to accompany your exercise session. The beat will help you keep to a rhythm while you work, and make the whole session more enjoyable.

Remember – if you don't use it, you lose it. So get your body working, and as soon as you start to see and feel the difference, you'll know it's been worth it.

Warm up

Start with a warm-up for the whole body to stimulate the circulation and firm up the back muscles.

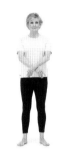

Have your feet hip-width apart and your toes pointing forwards. Cross your wrists in front of your body and pull in your tummy muscles. Lift your ribcage away from your waist – stand really tall, and keep your shoulders relaxed and down.

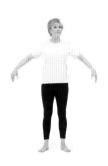

Take your arms out to your sides and circle them up.

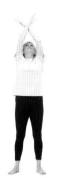

Cross them over your head (or as high as is comfortable) and back down in front of your body.

Get a good swing going and repeat 8 times, then reverse the direction 8 times.

Repeat the whole exercise twice more.

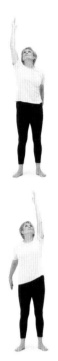

Stay in the same position and look straight ahead. Put one arm straight above your head, the other slightly behind you.

Move your arms forwards and back in a scissor movement for 10 beats, keeping your body still and relaxed.

Do one repeat of the circular movement, follow it with one repeat of the scissors, then shake out your arms to relax them.

Tummy Tightener

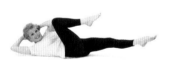

Lie flat on your back with your legs straight and your hands clasped behind your neck. Gently lift your shoulders off the ground – don't strain your neck – and keep your tummy pulled in and your mid and lower back in contact with the floor. Bring your right knee towards your chest until your leg forms a 45-degree angle to your body. At the same time raise your left leg slightly off the floor. Twist your left elbow towards your right knee.

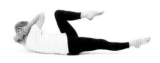

Come back to the centre, then straighten your right leg, bring your left knee up to your chest and twist your right elbow towards the left knee. You're making a 'cycling' movement with your legs and twisting your shoulders to touch alternate knees with your elbows, without putting your feet back on the floor.

Do 5 repetitions with each leg. Return to the resting position. Try to build up to 10 repetitions on each leg. If at any time you feel strain or pain in your lower back, stop at once.

Firm Up Your Tummy Muscles and Stretch Your Spine

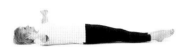

Lie on your back with your arms out at your sides in a crucifix position, palms facing upwards. Raise the arms so your hands are about 12 cm off the floor. Press your spine well into the floor to give you strength and stability.

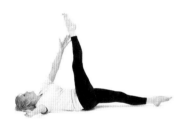

Lift your right leg straight up so that it forms a 45-degree angle with your body. At the same time, move your left hand across to touch your right foot. Count 2 beats to go up, then 2 beats to go down. Return your leg to the floor, but keep your hands suspended 12 cm above the ground.

Repeat 4 times.

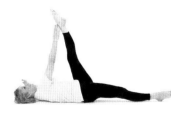

Then reverse, lifting the left leg and right arm.

Repeat 4 times.

Rest for 5 seconds, then repeat the exercise again on both sides.

Firm Up Your Outer Thighs and Strengthen Your Tummy Muscles

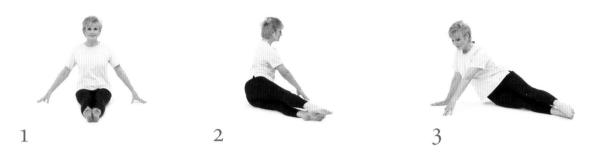

1   2   3

1   Sit on the floor with your legs together and your toes softly pointed. Your back should be straight and your fingertips resting gently on the floor beside you.
2   Roll over onto your left side, swinging your right arm over so it touches the floor on the left.
3   Then swing your left arm across and touch the floor on the right. You should feel you are rocking and rolling from side to side. Keep your legs straight and together.

Do 8 repetitions.

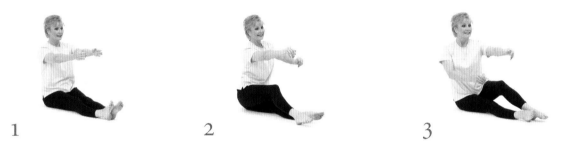

1   2   3

1   Then get ready to do bum walking across the floor.
2   Swing your hips and arms as you move and 'walk' your hips and bottom forwards across the floor for 8 counts.
Repeat the rocks and rolls above, then...
3   'Walk' backwards on your bottom for 8 counts.
Take a 5-second breather, then repeat the whole routine.

In other words, do a total of 8 rocks and rolls, 8 forward bum walks, 8 rocks and rolls and 8 reverse bum walks.

Firm Up Your Thighs and Tummy and Tone Your Legs

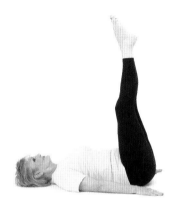

Lie on your back with your arms by your sides and your hands flat on the floor. Raise both legs straight up in the air to a 45-degree angle with your body.

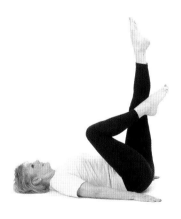

Bend one knee, keeping the other leg straight. Now gently 'air' cycle at a slow, steady beat for 8 counts with each leg. Then double up the speed for 16 counts.

Repeat a slow cycle for 8 counts, then double up again.

Tone Up Your Thighs, Upper Arms and Tummy

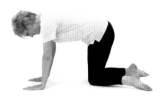

Kneel on all fours with your knees together and your hands flat on the floor, one under each shoulder. Keep the head and neck in line with the spine and don't drop towards the floor.

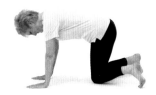

Keep your knees together and move your feet apart, taking them as wide as they can go.

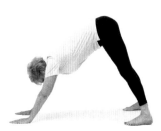

Curl your toes under, and slowly push up onto the balls of your feet with your legs beautifully straight. Lower your heels.

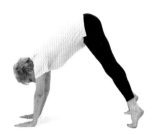

Then push back up onto your toes, lower down onto your heels again, push up onto the toes, then return to the kneeling position. Do 4 repetitions.

Rest for a few seconds.

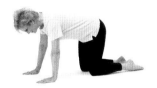

Now, remain kneeling on all fours, with your knees apart and your arms straight, your hands under your shoulders. Raise your head until it's level with your spine.

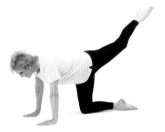

Straighten your left leg behind you, lifting it as high as it will go, and really stretch it out.

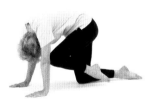

Swing it back in towards your body as if you are aiming to get your knee to touch your nose, then swing the leg back out again, keeping it nice and straight. Keep your back straight. Repeat for 8 counts. On the eighth backward swing, hold the leg in the air for a count of 3, then return to the kneeling position. Rest for a few seconds, then repeat the exercise with the right leg.

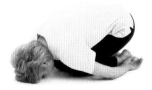

Bring your knees together and let the whole of your body sink back onto your heels. Rest your forehead on the floor, bring your arms back to the sides of your body, and relax.

If you find this too difficult, just sit back gently on your heels and relax your whole body.

Firm Up Your Bust and the Flab On the Upper Arms

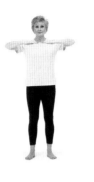

Stand with your feet hip-width apart and your toes pointing forwards. Raise your arms so they are level with your shoulders, bend them at the elbows and have your palms facing down.

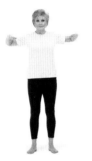

Pump your elbows behind you, keeping the arms bent, for 3 counts.

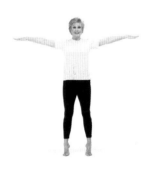

On the fourth count open your arms wide, stretching them back as far as they'll go, really opening up your chest. At the same time, lift your heels off the ground.

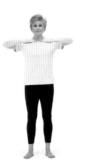

Return to the starting position.

It's most important during this exercise to keep your back strong and upright. Keep your tummy pulled in, and lift your ribcage.

Repeat 4 times.

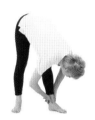

Drop your arms to your sides, then bend forwards and try to touch your left ankle with both hands.

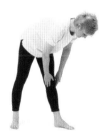

If you can't quite reach the ankle, touch either your knee or the side of your leg.

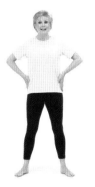

Straighten up and tap the sides of your body, then bend and repeat on the right side. By tapping first your ankle (or leg) then your sides, you'll get a nice rhythm going which will help with the timing of the exercise.

Repeat 8 times. Don't try this exercise if you are at all unsteady on your feet.

Then repeat the whole sequence once more.

Tone the Muscles of the Neck

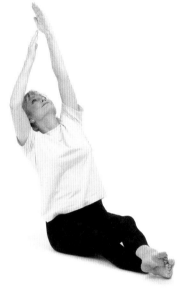

Sit on the floor with one leg crossed over the other at the ankles so you feel comfortable and relaxed. Place your hands very lightly on the floor beside you. Your back should be nice and straight. Look straight ahead.

Bring your right arm up and over your head, reaching as high as you can. At the same time look at your hand, feeling a long stretch in your neck. Now bring your left arm up, and again reach for the sky, looking at your left hand.

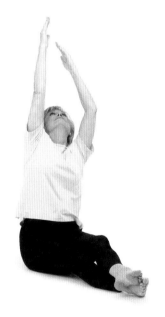

Now gently and alternately stretch your arms up as far as you can reach. This will cause you to make a small rocking movement from side to side with your shoulders as you give your arms a long, long, strong stretch and open up the spine. Reach as if your life depended on your touching the ceiling. Keep looking at your hands and feel the stretch in the neck muscles. You can also do this exercise sitting in a chair or standing up.

Do 8 repetitions – 4 on each side – then return to the starting position with your hands on the floor.

Give yourself a rest, then repeat once more.

Stretch Your Back and Tone the Hamstrings in Your Legs

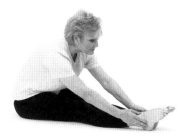

Sit on the floor, with your legs straight out in front of you and your back nice and straight. Have your hands at your sides. Gently lean forwards and put your hands on either side of your knees. Then, if you can, lean further forwards and place your hands on either side of your calves or your ankles.

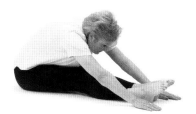

If you can, reach a little further forwards and rest your hands on the floor by your feet.

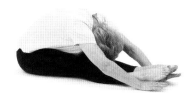

If you are really feeling strong and supple, lean even further forward and gently put your head on your legs and stretch your arms forward as far as they will go.

Gently uncurl and return to the sitting position.

If your back is not supple enough to go all the way down, don't strain. Go as far as you can, and after a few weeks, you'll find that you can reach even further with every session.

Do 4 repetitions.

Rest for a count of 5, then do another 4 repetitions.

Tighten Your Inner and Outer Thighs and Stretch Your Waist

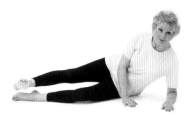

Lie on your left side with your left forearm resting on the ground propping up your body. Keep your left elbow well underneath your left shoulder. Your right arm is going to be your stabilizer. Place your right hand, flat on the floor, in front of your left hip. Slightly bend the left leg, but keep your right leg absolutely straight with your foot at a 45–degree angle and your toes pointing towards you.

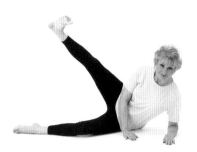

Raise your right leg towards your head, keeping it straight and with your toes still facing you.

Lower the leg down towards the right hand, lift it up again and lower it back down to the starting position. Keep your tummy firm during the exercise, it will help balance you and make sure you get maximum benefit from the lifts.

Take the exercise at a slow, controlled pace, and repeat 4 times.

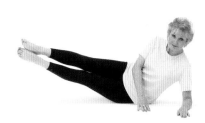

For a stronger and very advanced version of the same exercise, keep your body in the same position, on your left side with your right hand to stabilize you. Straighten both legs and lock them together. Gently lift both legs off the ground, still keeping them together. Hold for a count of one, then lower. You'll feel the stretch in your waist as well as in the thigh muscles.

Repeat 4 times.

Turn over and repeat the exercises on your right side using your left leg.

Strengthen Your Back and Tighten Your Bum

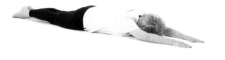

Lie on your tummy with your arms stretched straight out in front of you.

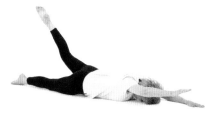

Raise your right arm and left leg at the same time, then return to the ground.

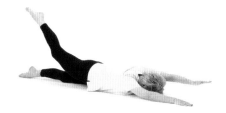

Raise the left arm and right leg.

Take it gently, control the movement and do 2 lifts on each side.

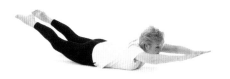

To continue and advance the exercise, lift both arms and legs together, raising your head off the ground as you bring up your arms for a slow count of 2.

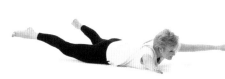

If you feel your back is strong enough, open your arms and legs as far as they will go so that your body looks like an X. Close, and return to the floor.

If you can't manage to spreadeagle your arms and legs, just do the lift and return to the floor, and rest your forehead back on the ground.

Do 2 repetitions.

Flabby Upper Arms

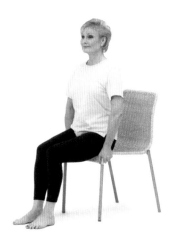

Place a hard-backed chair against a wall so it's secure and won't slide away. Sit on the edge of the chair, with the feet firmly on the ground, your back straight, tummy tight, and your arms holding on to the edge of the chair beside your thighs.

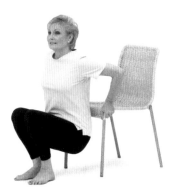

Taking your weight on your arms, gently ease yourself off the chair and lower your bottom so you are in a squatting position, bending your arms.

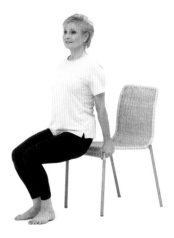

Then push up so the arms are straight, and lower again into a 'squat' position.

Do 10 repetitions, then sit back on the chair.
Take a short break, then repeat.

Cool Down

After any workout it's important to cool down and give your muscles, and your body, a chance to relax.

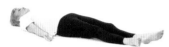

Lie flat on the floor, completely relaxed with your head to one side. Breathe slowly and deeply.

Bring your head to the centre, stretching out your spine, and close your eyes.

Breathe in deeply through your nose, feeling your lungs expand.

Hold for 3 seconds, then exhale through your mouth, totally emptying your lungs.

Repeat 3 times.

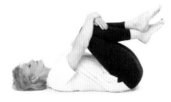

Slowly draw your knees up towards your chest, wrap your arms around them and gently rock from side to side to massage the whole of your spine and back.

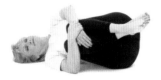

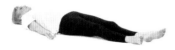

When you're ready, return your feet to the floor, lie back and just relax. Now have another drink of water!

Hands

If your hands are at all arthritic you must exercise them to strengthen the muscles around the affected joints or the pain will get worse. Every joint in the hand has muscles connected to it. By keeping those muscles strong and flexible they will support the joint, help it move and reduce your pain levels. Knitting, crotchet work, petit point, typing and sewing will all help keep your fingers agile and strong, as will these exercises.

Squeeze a tennis ball or an orange with one hand and try to make your fingers and thumb meet over the top of the ball. The exercise needs to be slow and controlled to get the maximum benefit.

Do 10 repetitions with each hand.

This exercise also helps increase bone density in the wrist.

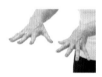

Do a Tommy Cooper. Throw your fingers out into a fully spread position, 'just like that!' Don't flick, make it slow and controlled. Really push them and try to hold your fingers extended for 5 seconds.

Do 5 repetitions with each hand.

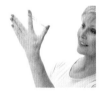

Elastic bands looped over your thumb and fingers will act like mini-exercise bands and strengthen the muscles. Loop the bands over your thumb, and over each finger individually. Stretch your fingers against the pressure of the band.

Work up to 10 repetitions on each finger.

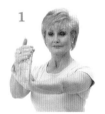 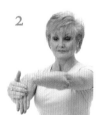 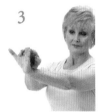 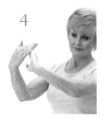

Flex your wrists. Using the fingers of your right hand, 1 push against the fingers of the left and push the wrist back, then 2 forwards, then 3 and 4 from side to side.
 Repeat on the other hand.

Knees

Painful, stiff knees need a two-pronged attack. First strengthen the muscles around the knee to give the joint support, then you can work on the mobilization of the joint itself.

Strengthening

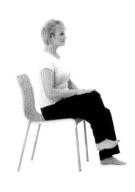

You can strengthen the the quadriceps on either side of the knee joints and give them support with a simple exercise that can be done sitting down so there is no weight on the joint.

Lift your foot about 3 cm off the ground and use your muscles to hold the leg and knee in that position for a count of 5.

Place your foot back on the floor, and lift it again almost immediately to repeat.

Start with 5 repetitions for a count of 5, and work up to 10 repetitions for a count of 10.

Remember to breathe! It's easy when you're doing this to concentrate so hard on the exercise that you hold your breath. Breathe deeply and slowly for maximum effect.

Controlled Squats

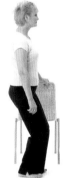

These can be done once the muscles start to strengthen, and provided there is not too much pain in the joints.

Hold on to a chair for support with your feet hip-width apart. Keeping your body upright, gently bend the knees to a point where you can still see your toes (look quickly and try not to tilt forwards or you will throw yourself off balance).

Hold the 'squat' for a count of 5, then return to the upright position.

Do 5 repetitions a day.

Improve Mobility and Reduce Pain

Good old-fashioned 'air' cycling is one of the best exercises. It moves the joint without putting any weight or strain on it. At home, try it in the bath where the water will give you extra support, or lie flat on your back on a nice warm, comfortable bed.

Gently cycle your knees, one leg at a time, so you don't put undue strain on your back, for about 30 seconds (it's longer than you think) and try to work up to a minute a day.

If you have access to a swimming pool, that's the best possible place to do any joint exercise because the water supports you and makes the muscles work even more efficiently.

 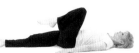 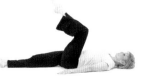 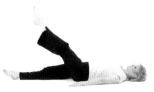

Hip Replacements

The most important thing to remember about hip-replacement operations is that they need time to settle and heal. For six months you should not do anything to disturb the new joint and only do any exercises given to you by your physiotherapist. But after that the muscles around the joint need to be stabilized and strengthened to give you back your mobility. If you do these exercises four to six weeks *before* the operation you'll be well on your way to a stronger hip joint and a quicker recovery after the procedure.

Leg Swings

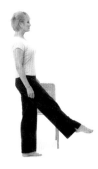

To strengthen the outer muscles, hold on to something solid like a sink, or the back of a chair (push it against a wall to give it stability). Keep your tummy muscles tight.

Gently swing the leg forwards and hold for a count of 5, then swing it backwards and hold for a count of 5. Next swing the leg out to the side, and again hold for a count of 5.

Do what feels comfortable, but aim for 5 complete repetitions.

Leg Squeezes

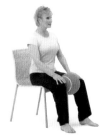

To strengthen the inner thigh muscles sit on the edge of a chair (again push it up to a wall to give it stability) and place a ball, a football or a beachball, or a pillow, between your knees.

Squeeze in and hold for 5. Do 5 repetitions.

Floor Work

This is essential for people who have had hip replacements because any exercise done on the floor will reduce the impact of gravity on the joints, and double the effect of the muscular activity. Floor work will also give your hip the correct alignment for exercise and ensure you start to get the full range of mobility in the joint.

1 Lie on the floor on your side, bend your lower leg and prop yourself up on your elbow to support the weight of your body. If your balance is a little unsteady, support yourself under the shoulder with a pillow.

2 Gently lift the top leg, slightly bent, as high as is comfortable. Hold it for 5 seconds, and then return to the floor. Repeat 5 times.

Do this exercise on both sides of the body so the muscles build equally on both hips. There's a great temptation to let your good hip do all the work. Resist it. It will throw your body out of alignment and encourage the muscles around the false hip to waste away.

1

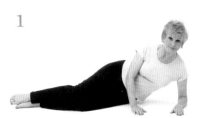

2

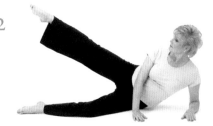

Feet

Most problems with feet stem from poor circulation and weak muscles (see Chapter Six). A great many problems can be eased with exercises that strengthen the muscles of the feet and make them more flexible.

A Simple Exercise

While sitting, put the feet flat on the floor and raise your toes so that only your heels are in contact with the floor. Push up as hard as you can. Return to the floor and raise your heels so that only your toes are in contact with the floor. Do 5 repetitions.

Tougher But More Effective

In a standing position, hold on to the sink or a chair. Raise yourself up on your toes so they are taking the whole weight of your body and hold for a count of 5. Keep your tummy muscles tight. Drop back down onto flat feet. Repeat 5 times.

Still holding on to the sink or a chair, raise your toes and balance on your heels. Hold for a count of 5. Repeat 5 times.

If you feel really strong walk on your toes, and then walk on your heels. This will really strengthen your feet, and is an excellent exercise for balance because you are taking the whole weight of your body on two tiny points.

Ankles

Can be strengthened and circulation improved with an exercise that needs you to be sitting on the edge of a chair with your shoes off. Clamp your knees, and put your feet

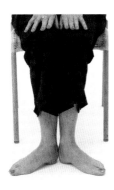 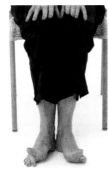

together. Then, keeping your heels together, move your big toes apart, keeping them in contact with the floor, until you form a 'V' shape with your feet.

Then, still keeping your heels together, bring your feet back to the centre by brushing your small toes against the floor.

Do this just a couple of times to start with, but work up to 5 repetitions a day and you'll see a marked improvement in your circulation and in the flexibility of your ankles.

Stiff Necks

A major warning: do not attempt to do a full neck roll by throwing your head back and 'rolling' in a complete circle unless you have a particularly flexible spine and have been exercising your neck for most of your life. Many mature people have a degree of arthritis in the upper spine and the muscles in the neck will not be sufficiently flexible to allow you to complete such a wide range of movement. It's possible, by putting your head back, to temporarily cut off the blood supply to your brain, and either become dizzy, or even pass out. That's often the reason for elderly people fainting in a supermarket, when they've put their head back to look at something on a top shelf.

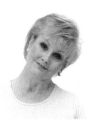

Side Bends

These will keep the neck supple. Take your ear towards your shoulder.
Keep your shoulder still so you don't bring your shoulder up to your ear!

Done slowly and in a gentle controlled movement, a couple of stretches a day should be enough.

Half Neck Rolls

These are OK if you just go from ear to ear, starting on the left side (1), and dropping the head forward (2), and round (3), until your right ear is over your right shoulder (4) – then repeating in the opposite direction.

If you feel you really must roll your head backwards, start by placing your hand at the top of your spine to support it, and roll your head gently back over your hand.

Do one roll in each direction.

1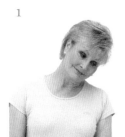

2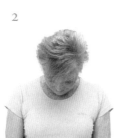

3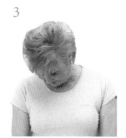

4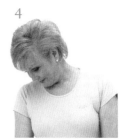

Stiff Shoulders

Shoulder Rolls

Keeping your hands by your side, roll your shoulders backwards in a circular movement for a count of 10, then forwards for a count of 10.

Keep your hands still so that only the shoulder muscles move in isolation without any help from the arms. Make the movements as controlled and as large as possible.

Shoulder Stretch

Lie flat on your back on the floor or sit in a chair and clasp your fingers together lightly, in front of you.

Swing your arms up and over your head, and if you are lying on the floor try to place your hands gently on the floor behind you. If you're sitting in a chair, go as far as you can. If you can't reach the floor, don't worry, after a few weeks you'll be able to. Push slightly to increase the stretch, and hold for a count of 5. Return your hands to your lap.

Repeat 3 times.

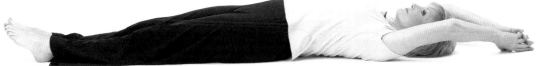

Circulation

If you have poor circulation and are worried about deep vein thrombosis (DVT) because you're sitting down a lot during the day, or are going on a long flight, there are several exercises you can do, in a chair (or plane seat) to keep your circulation active.

Legs and Feet

Both will benefit from the simple act of raising your toes as high as they'll go while keeping your feet on the ground, then reversing the action and raising your heels with your toes on the ground. Done 10 times it will keep the blood pumping, as will circling the ankles, first clockwise then anti-clockwise.

Bum Walking

This is usually done across the floor, but can be just as effective done on the spot in a seat. Move the buttocks as if they were 'walking' across the floor. Do 10 forwards and 10 backwards – but make sure you are on a firm chair that will not tip forwards.

Weak, Stiff Backs

It's amazing the amount of exercise you can do in a chair, so if you have limited mobility, or you just like exercising while watching television, the chair is a good place to start to strengthen your back.

Strengthening

Use a dyna band (available in most sports shops) or a pair of tights. Sit well back in the chair so your back is supported.

1 Put your arms out in front of you, shoulder-width apart, tighten your tummy muscles and pull against the exercise band (or tights) 2. When you've reached what you think is a full extension, bring your arms in towards your belly button 3, and pull apart on the band again 4.

Repeat 5 to 10 times.

As your strength improves, move forward from the back of the chair and keep good upright posture during the exercise.

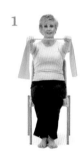

1

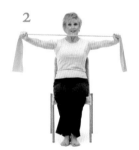

2

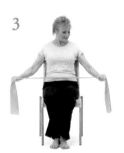

3

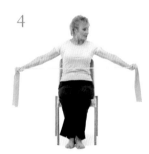

4

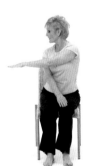

Improving Back Flexibility

Still sitting in the chair, place your right hand on your left knee, then take your left arm around the front of your body at shoulder height.

Now, keeping the elbow slightly bent and still at shoulder height, gently take your right arm behind you towards the back of the chair. You'll feel a twist in your spine. Don't let your hips move.

Repeat on the other side.

Do 5 repetitions on each side.

Crawling on All Fours

Providing you don't have sore knees, this is really good for strengthening not just your back, but also your wrists, and it helps with balance too. Try sideways and backwards crawling – if these are more difficult then all the more reason to practise.

The Cobra

This is a yoga position which, when done gently, will really help to strengthen and loosen a stiff spine.

Lie on the floor on your tummy. Place your hands under your shoulders, tighten your tummy muscles and gently lift your shoulders and upper body off the floor, using your back muscles. Keep your hips and feet on the ground.

If you have a really stiff back you may only be able to manage a couple of centimetres, if anything at all, to start with. But persevere. Go gently, and stop if you feel any pain.

Do 2 repetitions and hold for a count of 4.

Chair Bouncing – A Good All Round Exercise

This is a really good exercise that uses a whole range of muscles in the body, and can be done easily at home without any equipment other than a dining chair.

1 Sit on the edge of a chair with your feet about 10 cm apart and your toes slightly back from your knees. 2 Place your hands on your knees and rise out of the chair just a few inches, pause, then 3 rise a little higher, pause and 4 rise a little higher again, then lower your rear as if you are about to sit down. Only don't sit down, but repeat the exercise.

It must be slow and controlled, and if you can keep that up for a minute – or 5 to 10 repetitions – your muscles will be screaming, and you'll be giving yourself an incredibly strengthening workout that benefits your knees, legs, hips, stomach, ankles and back.

If you have sore knees you may want to put a pillow on the chair so you are starting higher and not putting as much pressure on your knees.

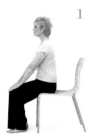
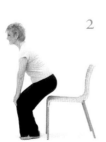
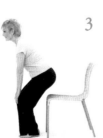
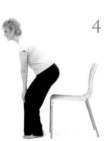

Diabetes

Exercises that improve your strength and endurance will help to increase the insulin sensitivity of your muscles, and do wonders for your circulation.

High Blood Pressure

In 1993 the World Health Organisation (WHO) recommended that in many cases a combination of a sensible diet and regular exercise would do more to reduce hypertension and high blood pressure than a course of pills. As high blood pressure is one of the major causes of stroke, if you're not already doing some form of regular exercise programme, it's worth starting gently by looking at a course of yoga, Pilates, or t'ai chi, or taking up swimming. A brisk thirty-minute walk three times a week is also a great stress buster.

Pelvic Floor Muscles

A combination of childbearing and age tends to make a woman's pelvic floor muscles weaken in later years. (It is also an increasing problem in men.) Loss of bladder control means that sneezing or coughing can make you lose water involuntarily, and no matter how well you might control the urge to go to the toilet, the minute you put the key in the door, you know the floodgates are going to open. Exercising the muscles will not only improve control, it should also sharpen up your sex life and reduce the risk of urinary infection because of dryness. There's also some evidence to show that in older women a bladder infection can affect their balance, so keeping the pelvic floor muscles strong will not only control the flow of urine, but also protect against infection.

The pelvic floor muscle is the one you contract when you want to stop the flow of urine. If your muscles are working well you should be able to stop the flow at any stage. If not then you need help. Most of the large chemist chains sell pelvic floor weights which ensure you use the right muscles to grip and hold them in place. They're very easy to use, and you can do the exercises while doing the housework, or putting on your make-up. Or you can try this simple exercise.

Contract the muscle rapidly for a count of 5 beats and then hold contracted on the fifth beat for 5 seconds. Do 10 repetitions daily. Ensure you isolate the muscle when you exercise so that you don't contract the stomach instead. You can do while it sitting down watching television, in the car, at the bus stop or even in the supermarket checkout. It's such a discreet and private exercise, no one will know you're doing it. Unless, that is, they guess something's up from the slight smile on your face!

My top ten must haves

1 Liz Earle's Cleanse and Polish
2 Moisturizer
3 Body lotion
4 Body brush
5 Foot file
6 Nail file
7 A bottle of still water
8 Cod liver oil capsules
9 Heated curling tongs
10 Vaseline

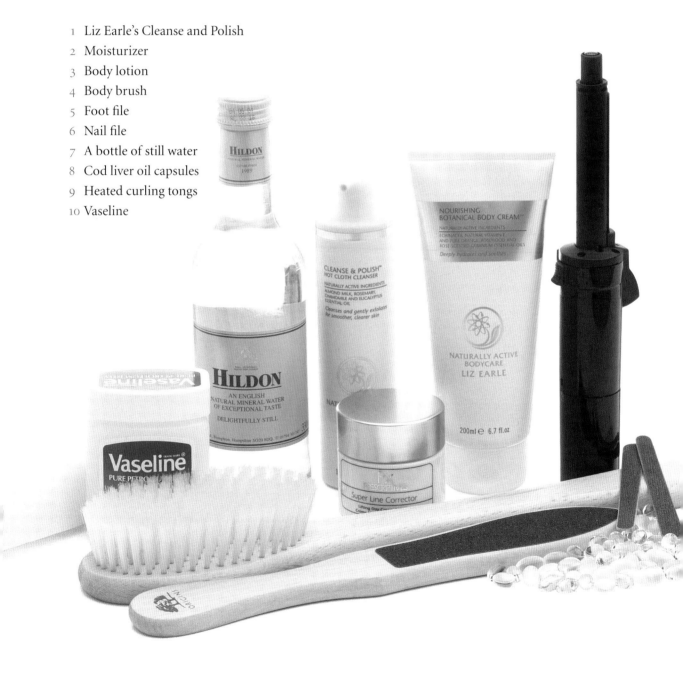

Useful Names and Addresses

Age Concern
Astral House
1268 London Road
London SW16 4ER
TEL 0800 009966
WEB www.ageconcern.org.uk

Alzheimer's Society
Gordon House
10 Greencoat Place
London SW1P 1PH
TEL *Helpline* 0845 300 0336
      Mon–Fri 8.30 a.m. to 6.30 p.m.
WEB www.alzheimers.org.uk

The Amarant Trust
Head Office
The Amarant Centre
Gainsborough Clinic
80 Lambeth Road
London SE1 7PW
TEL 020 7401 3855
WEB www.amarantmenopausetrust.
      org.uk
Special advice line manned by menopause
nurses Mon–Fri from 11 a.m to 6 p.m.
01293 413 000

The Arthritic Association
First Floor Suite
2 Hyde Gardens
Eastbourne
East Sussex BN21 1AA
TEL 01323 416 550 and 020 7491 0233
WEB www.arthriticassociation.org.uk

ASH
(*Action on Smoking and Health*)
102 Clifton Street
London EC2A 4HW
WEB www.ash.org.uk

Association of Reflexologists
27 Old Gloucester Street
London WC1N 3XX
TEL 0870 567 3320
WEB www.aor.org.uk
Send a 44p SAE for a full list of all
registered practitioners

BackCare
16 Elmtree Road
Teddington
Middlesex TW11 8ST
TEL 020 8977 5474
WEB www.backcare.org.uk

Barielle
TEL 020 7636 0234
WEB www.barielle.co.uk

Blood Pressure Association
60 Cranmer Terrace
London SW17 0QS
TEL 020 8772 4994
WEB www.bpassoc.org.uk

British Acupuncture Council
53 Jeddo Road
London W2 9HQ
TEL 020 8735 0400
WEB www.acupuncture.org.uk

British Association of Aesthetic
Plastic Surgeons
The Royal College of Surgeons
35–43 Lincoln's Inn Fields
London WC2A 3PE
TEL 020 7405 2234
WEB www.baaps.org.uk

British Dance Council
Terpsichore House
240 Merton Road
South Wimbledon
London SW19 1EQ
TEL 020 8545 0085
Send an SAE and they will enclose details
of all dance clases, ballroom, Latin and
Western, in your area
WEB www.british-dance-council.org

British Dental Association
64 Wimpole Street
London W1E 8YS
TEL *Word of Mouth Helpline* 0870 333 118

British Heart Foundation
14 Fitzhardinge Street
London W1H 6DH
TEL 020 7935 0185
WEB www.bhf.org.uk

British Menopause Society
4–6 Eton Place
Marlow
Bucks SK7 2QA
TEL 01628 890199

British Wheel of Yoga
25 Jermyn Street
Sleaford
Lincs NG34 7RU
TEL   01529 306 851
WEB   www.bwy.org.uk

CancerBACUP
3 Bath Place
Rivington Street
London EC2A 3JR
TEL   freephone 0808 800 1234,
Mon–Fri 9 a.m. to 7 p.m.
WEB   www.cancerbacup.org.uk

Cancer Research UK
PO Box 123
London WC2A 3PX
TEL   020 7269 3662
WEB   www.cancerhelp.org.uk

Country and Western Dance Council
(Line Dancing)
TEL   01278 452 743

Diabetes UK
10 Parkway
London NW1 7AA
TEL   020 7424 1000
WEB   www.diabetes.org.uk

Fitness League
52 London Street
Chertsey
Surrey KT16 8AJ
TEL   01932 564 567
WEB   www.thefitnessleague.com

Help the Aged
207–221 Pentonville Road
London N1 9UZ
TEL   020 7278 1114
WEB   www.helptheaged.org.uk

The Keep Fit Association
Astra House
Suite 1.05
Arklow Road
London SE14 6EB
TEL   020 8692 9566
WEB   www.keepfit.org.uk

Liz Earle
Mail order telephone   01983 813913

National Osteoporosis Society
Camerton
Bath BA2 0PJ
TEL   01761 471771
WEB   www.nos.org.uk

NHS Smoking helpline
TEL   0800 169 0169
WEB   www.givingupsmoking.co.uk

The Patients Association
PO Box 935
Harrow
Middlesex HA1 3YJ
TEL   020 8423 9111
WEB   www.patients-association.com

Plastic Surgery Partners
55 Harley Street
London W1G 8QR
TEL   020 8735 6060
WEB   www.cosmeticsurgeryuk.com

QUIT
(help for people who want to stop
smoking)
Ground Floor
211 Old Street
London EC1V 9NR
TEL   020 7251 1551
         Quitline 0800 002200
WEB   www.quit.org.uk

The Stroke Association
Stroke House
240 City Road
London EC1V 2PR
TEL   0845 303 3100
WEB   www.stroke.org.uk

T'ai Chi Union of Great Britian
94, Felsham Road
London SW15 1DQ
TEL   020 8788 9130

Useful books

Yoga
Barbara Currie, *Fabulous Shape Forever*, Chameleon, 2002.

Pilates
Lynne Robinson and Caroline Brien, *The Perfect Body the Pilates Way*,
Macmillan, 1997.

Index